Health Essentials

Reflexology

Inge Dougans was born in Denmark where she also received her reflexology training. In 1981 she moved to South Africa where she set up her own clinic. In 1983 she started the School of Reflexology and Meridian Therapy and in 1985 she formed the South African Reflexology Society. She gives lectures and workshops on Reflexology throughout the UK, Europe and USA and runs a busy practice in South Africa.

Suzanne Ellis was born in South Africa. She obtained an English degree from the University of Natal and has worked as a Journalist, documentary script-writer and magazine editor. She trained as a reflexologist with Inge Dougans.

The Health Essentials Series

There is a growing number of people who find themselves attracted to holistic or alternative therapies and natural approaches to maintaining optimum health and vitality. The *Health Essentials* series is designed to help the newcomer by presenting high quality introductions to all the main complementary health subjects. Each book presents all the essential information on each therapy, explaining what it is, how it works and what it can do for the reader. Advice is also given, where possible, on how to begin using the therapy at home, together with comprehensive lists of courses and classes available worldwide.

The *Health Essentials* titles are all written by practising experts in their fields. Exceptionally clear and concise, each text is supported by attractive illustrations.

Series Medical Consultant
Dr John Cosh, MD, FRCP

In the same series

Acupuncture by Peter Mole
Alexander Technique by Richard Brennan
Aromatherapy by Christine Wildwood
Ayurveda by Scott Gerson MD
Chi Kung by James MacRitchie
Chinese Medicine by Tom Williams
Colour Therapy by Pauline Wills
Flower Remedies by Christine Wildwood
Herbal Medicine by Vicki Pitman
Kinesiology by Ann Holdway
Massage by Stewart Mitchell
Shiatsu by Elaine Liechti
Skin and Body Care by Sidra Shaukat
Spiritual Healing by Jack Angelo
Vitamin Guide by Hasnain Walji

Health Essentials

REFLEXOLOGY

Foot Massage
for Total Health

Inge Dougans

with

Suzanne Ellis

ELEMENT
Shaftesbury, Dorset ● Rockport, Massachusetts
Brisbane, Queensland

© Inge Dougans 1991

First published in Great Britain in 1991 by
Element Books Limited
Shaftesbury, Dorset SP7 8BP

Published in the USA in 1991 by
Element Books, Inc.
42 Broadway, Rockport, MA 01966

Reprinted January and December 1992
Reprinted 1993
Reprinted March and October 1994
Reprinted 1995

Published in Australia in 1993 by
Element Books Limited for
Jacaranda Wiley Limited
33 Park Road, Milton, Brisbane 4064

Cover design by Max Fairbrother
Designed by Nancy Lawrence
Typeset in Goudy by Selectmove Limited.
Printed and bound in Great Britain by
Biddles Ltd, Guildford & King's Lynn

British Library Cataloguing in Publication Data
Dougans, Inge
Health Essentials: reflexology.
I. Title II. Ellis, Suzanne
615.822

ISBN 1–85230–218–6

Note from the Publisher

Any information given in any book in the *Health Essentials* series is not
intended to be taken as a replacement for medical advice. Any person
with a condition requiring medical attention should consult a qualified
medical practitioner or suitable therapist.

Contents

I would like to dedicate this book to all the students of reflexology, past, present and future. Without them, this practice could never have evolved into the respected and effective healing art it is today.

Author's special note: Throughout this book, the term 'foot massage' is used as a convenient shorthand to describe Reflexology. However, the authors would stress that this is a convenience term only and is not a proper technical description of the therapy. Reflexology is not massage as understood in the systematic and scientific manipulation of the soft tissues of the body. Reflexology is the application of specific pressures to reflex points in the hands and feet.Nevertheless we feel massage is a useful shorthand justified in this instance for a general understanding of what is involved.

1

What is Reflexology?

REFLEXOLOGY IS A gentle art, a fascinating science and an extremely effective form of therapeutic foot massage. This therapy falls into the realm of 'complementary' medicine. As such, reflexology is considered to be a holistic healing technique which aims to treat the individual as a whole, in order to induce a state of balance and harmony in body, mind and spirit.

Since the time of Hippocrates, health has been defined as a balanced state, and disease an imbalanced state. In modern society, imbalance is the norm. We speed our way through life as if there were no tomorrow, and the demands of the high-speed twentieth century techno-generation are taking their toll on the delicate and intricate human body. A majority of people teeter on the edge of ill-health – in a state of dis-ease and imbalance – and find it difficult to cope with the stresses of day-to-day life. Their potential for perfect health is shrouded by various negative influences. But this potential is in each and every one of us; all it needs as a starting point is the desire to reach a balanced state, which will enable us to enjoy continuous health and vitality. The transition from the state of imbalance to a balanced state requires a gentle and harmless healing process – a process seldom found in the dangerous drugs and radical surgery sometimes so indiscriminately prescribed us by the practitioners of conventional medicine.

Many of the ills of modern man cannot be cured by artificial drugs – drugs more inclined to damage and suppress than to heal. The body heals itself – if given the chance. Because this healing power lies within, we should learn to support and nurture it, not suppress it. Reflexology helps us do this by activating the body's natural healing powers and working to re-establish the equilibrium necessary for normal functioning.

Few people are aware of the fundamental role of feet in health and healing. In fact, few people pay any attention to their feet at all. We tend to torture and neglect them . . . we squeeze them into ill-fitting fashionable shoes, suffocate them in socks and stockings, pound pavements, hike trails and altogether place an inordinate amount of strain on our poor feet. They bear our weight, cope with bad posture and generally take a severe beating on their path through life. Although we may be vaguely aware of the important role they play in carrying us through life, few realize the significant role of our feet in our spiritual and physical well-being.

Our feet connect us to the ground and they are therefore a connection between our earthly and spiritual life. They ground us literally and figuratively. They are our base and foundation and our contact with the earth and the energies that flow through it. And they can also play a major role in attaining and maintaining better health and well-being.

This is because the feet are a perfect microcosm of the body. All the organs, glands and other parts of the body are laid out in the same arrangement on the feet as 'reflections/reflexes' of the body parts. A reflex is an involuntary or unconscious response to a stimulus. In reflexology, when the reflexes on the feet are stimulated, an involuntary response is elicited in organs and glands connected by energy pathways to these specific reflexes. These reflexes, when correctly stimulated, can have a profound influence on our state of health.

This microcosmic representation of body parts is also evident in the iris of the eye, in the ear and on the hands. These representations of body parts are, however, easiest to locate on the feet, where they cover a larger area and are more specific; this makes them easy to work with. The feet are also particularly sensitive, due to the abundance of nerve endings present.

Nerves conduct electrical impulses. Imagine these impulses as channels of energy which connect the feet to the rest of the body. When pressure is applied to certain points on the feet, electro-chemical nerve impulses are activated, forming a 'message'. This message passes through 'afferent neurons' (neurons conveying messages to the centre) to a ganglion (a collection of nerve cells and fibres which form an independent nerve centre outside the spinal cord and the brain). The message then passes from the ganglion via 'efferent neurons' (conveying messages out from the centre to the periphery) to the specific organ, which will then respond. The nerve impulses initiated by pressing reflex areas on the feet might possibly link into the autonomic nervous system, which is primarily concerned with the involuntary action of internal organs, muscles and glands.

The goal of reflexology is to trigger the return to homoeostasis – a state of equilibrium or balance. The most important step towards achieving this is to reduce tension and induce relaxation. Relaxation is the first step to normalization. When the body is relaxed, circulation can flow unimpeded and supply nutrients and oxygen necessary to the cells, and the body organs can return to a normal state and function efficiently.

Professional massage of the reflex areas on the feet serves to establish which parts of the body are out of balance and therefore not working efficiently. Treatment can then be given to correct these imbalances and thus return the body to good working order. Not only is this form of therapy useful for treating ill-health, but it is also effective in maintaining good health and preventing illness. With reflex massage health problems can be detected early and treatment given to prevent serious symptoms from developing.

One of the most important benefits of reflexology is its efficacy in inducing a state of relaxation. Stress – a major problem of the twentieth century – is directly responsible for a multitude of modern diseases and disorders. Constant exposure to stress gradually erodes the body's immune system, and the end result is disease. Some estimates indicate that up to 90 per cent of modern diseases are a direct result of prolonged exposure to stress. Because reflexology reduces the negative effects of stress and helps the body normalize, it helps ward off the potential of more lethal disease.

HOW IT ALL BEGAN

Foot massage is not new to the human race. There is strong evidence that a form of foot therapy, similar to what we call reflexology today, has been practised for centuries by many diverse cultures around the world.

Exactly where it all began is still somewhat elusive. As yet, there is no conclusive proof that modern reflexology had its roots in ancient China, but the main school of thought claims that it originated in the East at about the same time as acupuncture. To quote Dr W. Fitzgerald in his book *Zone Therapy*:

A form of treatment by means of pressure points was known in India and China some 5000 years ago. This knowledge appears to have been lost and forgotten; perhaps it was set aside in favour of acupuncture which emerged as a stronger growth from the same root.

This view is also taken by Dr Franz Wagner (*Reflex Zone Massage*):

The ancient Chinese developed the technique of acupressure, the roots of which lie in the knowledge of reflex zones and the relationships between them. Today the most highly developed and perhaps strongest branch of this ancient form of therapy is acupuncture. In massaging the reflex zones of the feet we are massaging tissue, and we are working along the meridians of acupuncture.

Historically, the Chinese were way ahead of Westerners in understanding the holistic functioning of the human body and its relationship to external natural forces. Thousands of years ago they developed the idea that different parts of the body represent different contacts with the outside world: the head connects us to heaven; with our hands we contact each other by touching and working together; the nipples are the contact that binds us with nourishment to the world; the genitals carry new life that can be born into the world; the anus connects us to the world through the cycle of matter and the feet connect us to the earth through movement.

The Chinese were also aware of the importance of feet in treating disease. In AD 1017, Dr Wang Wei had a human figure cast in bronze on which were marked those points on the body important for acupuncture. When this knowledge was put into practice in treating the sick, the practitioner positioned the needles in the appropriate areas of the body and then applied deep pressure therapy on the soles of the inside and outside edge of both feet. Concentrated pressure was then applied on the big toe. The feet were used in conjunction with the acupuncture needles to channel extra energy through the body. Dr Wei said that the feet were the most sensitive part of the body and contained great energizing areas.

There can therefore be little doubt that a strong connection exists between reflexology and acupuncture. They are certainly based on similar ideas. Both are considered meridian therapies, which propose that energy lines link the hands and feet to various body parts. However, while acupuncture went from strength to strength in the East, reflexology was, for some unknown reason, disregarded. It has only recently re-emerged in the West. Acupuncture, despite its popularity in the East, was an unknown art in the West until introduced into western medicine in 1883, by Dutch physician Ten Tyne. Until the introduction of acupuncture to the West, western medicine did not acknowledge the meridian energy system – a system which plays a vital role in my approach to reflexology.

Apart from the Chinese, other ancient cultures also practised foot massage as a form of therapeutic and preventative medicine. The oldest documentation depicting the practice of reflexology was discovered in Egypt. This, a pictograph, is dated around 2500–2330 BC. It was found at Saqqara in the tomb of an Egyptian physician, Ankmahor. The scene in the pictograph depicts two darker skinned men 'working' on the feet of two men with lighter skin. Apparently the heiroglyphic above the scene reads: Patient: 'Do not hurt me.' Practitioner: 'I shall act so you praise me.'

Another theory claims that foot reflex therapy was passed down to the American Indians by the Incas. One American Indian tribe – the Cherokee Indians of North Carolina – can attest that they have, for centuries, acknowledged the importance of feet in maintaining physical, mental and spiritual balance. According to Jenny Wallace, a therapist from this clan:

In my tribe working on the feet is a very important healing art and is part of a sacred ceremony. The feet walk upon the earth and through this your spirit is connected to the universe. Our feet are our contact with the earth and the energies that flow through it.

Reflexology may have remained the property of these ancient and exotic cultures and been lost to the West had it not been for the enquiring medical minds in Europe and America in the late nineteenth and early twentieth centuries.

The Germans began to look at physiological reflex action in the late 1890s and early 1900s. They began to examine the treatment of disease by massage and developed techniques that became known as reflex massage. It is generally believed that Dr Alfons Cornelius was probably the first to apply massage to 'reflex zones'. The story goes that in 1893, Cornelius suffered an infection. In the course of his convalescence he received a daily massage. At the spa he noticed how effective the massages of one particular medical officer were. The man worked longer on areas that he found painful. This concept inspired Cornelius, who, after examining himself, instructed his masseur to work only on the painful areas. His pain quickly disappeared and in four weeks he had completely recovered. This led him to pursue the use of pressure in his own medical practice. He published his manuscript *Druckpunkte* or *Pressure Points* in 1902. However, American Dr William Fitzgerald is the person who deserves most credit for establishing the basis of modern reflexology with his 'discovery' of zones and his techniques known as 'zone therapy'.

ZONE THERAPY

Dr William Fitzgerald, regarded as the founder of zone therapy, was born in Connecticut, USA, in 1872. He graduated in medicine from the University of Vermont and spent two and a half years working at the Boston City Hospital. He also practised at hospitals in Vienna, and London. While working in Vienna, he probably came into contact with the work of Dr H. Bressler, who was investigating the possibility of treating organs with pressure points. Fitzgerald noticed that, when treating different patients for the same disorder with a minor operation, some would feel considerable pain while others would feel very little. His investigations revealed that those who experienced little pain were actually producing an anaesthetic effect on themselves by applying pressure to areas of their bodies. Intrigued by this, he continued his research into this phenomenon while he was working as Head Physician at the Hospital for Diseases of the Ear, Nose and Throat in Hartford, Connecticut, testing out many of his theories on patients. He found that if pressure was applied to the fingers, it would create an anaesthetic effect on the hand, arm and shoulder, right up to the jaw, face, ear and nose. He applied the pressure using tight bands of elastic on the middle section of each finger or with small clamps which he placed on the tips. He was able to carry out minor surgical operations just using this pressure technique. By exerting this pressure on a specific part of the body he learned to predict which other parts of the body would be affected.

Developing this work further, he systemized the body into zones. He established ten equal longitudinal zones running the length of the body from the top of the head to the tips of the toes. The number ten corresponds to the fingers and toes. Each finger and toe falls into one zone. To establish the zone divisions, imagine a line drawn through the centre of the body with five zones on either side of this line. The thumb and big toe fall into zone one and the small finger and toe both fall into zone five. These zones are of equal width and extend right through the body from front to back. The theory is that parts of the body found within a certain zone will be linked to one another by the energy flow within the zone and can therefore affect one another.

Fitzgerald and his colleague Dr Edwin Bowers were so enthusiastic about their discoveries that they developed a unique method of convincing colleagues of the validity of their theory. They would apply pressure to the sceptical person's hand, then stick a pin in the area of the face anaesthetized by the pressure. This was rather a dramatic way to prove a point, but it worked! In 1915, Bowers wrote the article that first publicly described this treatment which they had named 'zone therapy'. This was published in *Everybody's*

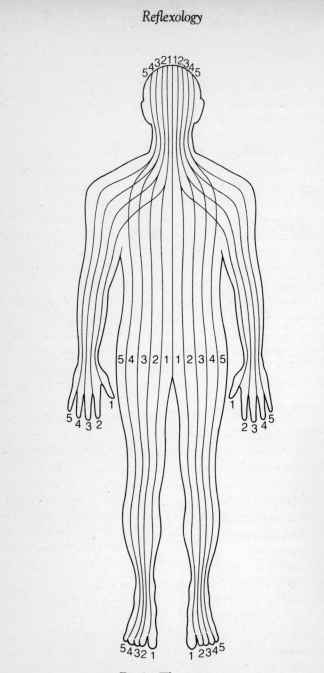

Fig. 1. The zones

Magazine and entitled 'To Stop That Toothache Squeeze Your Toe!'

In 1917, the combined work of Dr Fitzgerald and Dr Bowers was published in the book *Zone Therapy*. Diagrams of the zones of the feet and the corresponding division of the ten zones of the body appeared in the first edition of this book. The reflex areas, so crucial to modern reflexology, were not singled out for any special attention by Fitzgerald.

Fitzgerald and his theories were not enthusiastically received by the medical profession, but one physician believed in this work – Dr Joseph Riley. This was most auspicious, as it was Riley's research assistant Eunice Ingham who was destined to make the greatest contribution to modern reflexology.

Eunice Ingham (1879–1974) should probably be referred to as the Mother of Modern Reflexology. It was as a result of her untiring research and dedication that reflexology finally came into its own. She separated the work on the reflexes of the feet from zone therapy in general. Ingham had been using zone therapy in her work but began to feel more strongly that the feet should be specific targets for the therapy, because of their highly sensitive nature. She charted the feet in relation to the zones and their effects on the rest of the anatomy, until finally she had evolved on the feet themselves a 'map' of the entire body. So successful were her findings, and so effective her treatments, that her reputation soon spread. She took her work to the public and non-medical community as she realized that lay people could learn the proper reflexology techniques to help themselves, their families and friends. She was called on to speak at conventions and shared her knowledge with chiropodists, masseurs and physiotherapists, naturopaths and osteopaths. For over thirty years Eunice Ingham travelled America teaching her method through books, charts and seminars to thousands of people in and out of the medical profession. Her two books *Stories The Feet Can Tell* (1938) and *Stories The Feet Have Told* (1951) were probably the first books written on the subject. Today her legacy continues under the direction of her nephew Dwight Byers who runs the International Institute of Reflexology in St Petersburg.

Zone therapy is without doubt the basis of modern reflexology and most reflexologists use this as a useful adjunct to

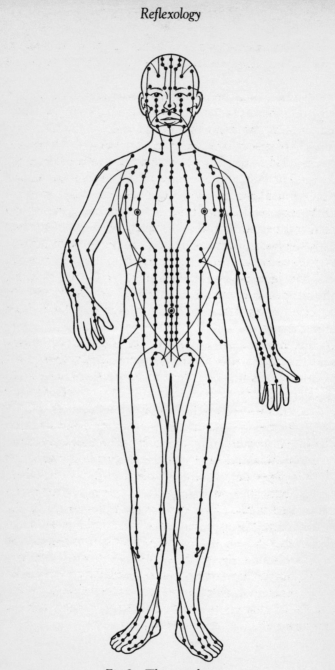

Fig. 2. The meridians

reflexology. However, it is my belief that the Chinese meridian system is, in fact, the vital link between the feet and the rest of the body.

The question as to the relationship between reflexology, acupuncture, shiatsu and acupressure is often asked. According to acupuncture, the body has twelve pairs of meridians or pathways. These form the single energy system and maintain the health of the organism. Meridians are pathways through which the energy of the universe circulates throughout the body organs and keeps the universe and the body in harmony. The acupuncturist believes that illness or pain occurs when the pathways become blocked, disrupting the energy flow and breaking the body's harmony. The Chinese, in acupuncture, developed the use of needles to unblock these pathways. In shiatsu, the Japanese use direct thumb and finger pressure on the acupuncture points to achieve similar results. In reflexology, finger pressure unblocks the sections of meridians found in the feet.

To date, most reflexologists have believed in the energy lines of the zone system. Although this theory has stood many reflexologists in good stead and contributed greatly to the development of modern reflexology, I personally do not adhere to this theory. I believe that the effects elicited by massaging the feet are caused by stimulation of the six main meridians that run through the feet. Fitzgerald recognized the energy connection between the feet and other body parts, and without his pioneering work, reflexology might not be where it is today. But as the eastern concept of energy systems was not recognized in the West at the time of his research, the connection with the meridians was not understood. I am convinced that the energy channels linking the feet to the other body parts are the meridians described by the Chinese in acupuncture, and not the zones described by Dr Fitzgerald. This book, therefore, differs from previous reflexology books, because we now move away from the theory of zone therapy and into the realm of meridian therapy.

2

What Can Reflexology Do For You?

REFLEXOLOGY IS A holistic therapy and as such, aims to treat the body as a whole, endeavouring to get to the root cause of disease and treat this – not the symptom. For best results the participation of the patient is required. In all holistic therapies, much emphasis is placed on taking responsibility for your own state of health. In orthodox medicine, the tendency is to hand over responsibility to the doctor and expect him to cure all ills. This is a bit of a tall order. Dis-ease is a direct result of your own thoughts and actions. In order to change this, you have to take a long hard look at yourself – something many people don't find easy. It is usually far more simple to place the responsibility and blame outside yourself. This attitude however, will rarely facilitate a true cure.

People venturing into the field of complementary medicine must understand that there is no such thing as an instant cure. Becoming well requires a healing process – a process which often not only affects the body, but the mind as well, bringing to the awareness the overwhelming effects that attitude, lifestyle and diet have on health. Once this is accepted, it becomes obvious that in order to achieve perfect health and well-being, we must be prepared to make an effort to substitute good habits for bad.

It is also imperative to be willing to 'let go' of disease. A reflexology practitioner will be compassionate, caring and dedicated to the client's welfare, but no practitioner can decide for the client that he/she is going to get well. That, the client has to do for himself. Many people hang on to disease as a psychological security blanket. We discover at a very early age that illness elicits sympathy and attention and all too often this conditioning stays with us into adulthood, and becomes a hard habit to break. A genuine desire for health and willingness to let go of disease is of vital importance to any healing process.

Reflexology is not a magic panacea or any kind of instant short-cut. The role of reflexology is to facilitate healing. The reflexologist doesn't cure – only the body cures. What reflexology does is work with the subtle energy flows which revitalize the body so that its own natural healing capacity can get to work. The specific techniques for applying pressure to the feet create channels for healing energy to circulate to all parts of the body.

The human body is a magnificent machine. Thousands of parts work together to keep the body functioning at optimum levels. Unfortunately, the negative effects of attitudes, lifestyle and diet throw the body out of sync, causing malfunctions in various parts. If one part ceases to function efficiently, the whole suffers. Then the minor aches, pains and general fatigue that are often forerunners of more serious complaints begin to manifest. The analogy of a car – a very good example – is often used. To get maximum response from your car, you have to keep it in good working order – if one part is out of order, the performance of the car suffers, and it has to go to the garage for a tune-up or you trade it in for a new one. Reflexology can be considered a body tune-up. And as you can't trade your body in for a new one, it makes good sense to look after the one you have!

So, what exactly can reflexology do for you? By far the most important benefit of reflexology is its ability to reduce stress and induce deep relaxation. When in a relaxed state, the body has the opportunity to heal itself and function more efficiently. Another positive effect is improved circulation. This in turn cleanses the body of toxins and impurities. Improved nerve supply, revitalized energy and overall body balancing are further positive effects.

As stress is one of the greatest problems in this last decade of the twentieth century, and the prime instigator of numerous more deadly diseases, it is in the role of stress reduction that reflexology can be of most benefit.

REFLEXOLOGY VERSUS THE STRESS SYNDROME

Stress is difficult to avoid. It is an integral part of modern life. The days when the stress syndrome was only associated with high-powered business executives are long gone. Today, young children, women, men and the elderly are all subject to varying degrees of stress. Survival in twentieth century society is stressful – traffic, television, noise, job pressure, family problems, financial problems; and global problems such as wars, famines, disease, environmental imbalances, pollution – the list is endless. Few escape the consequences of stress. The increasing number of people with high blood pressure, heart attacks and strokes is evidence of this – and these are only the more obvious stress-related diseases. Other symptoms are more nebulous. Long-term symptoms of constant exposure to stress are fatigue, anxiety and depression. The nervous system becomes so drained and depleted that the only physical reaction is fatigue.

Not all stress is negative. It can be immensely stimulating. An athlete or performer subjects himself to the stress which is part of achieving and experiencing life's ultimate sensations. The human body is equipped to cope with this kind of short-term stress. But long-term, constant exposure to stress is devastating. Persistent daily stresses gradually erode the body's immune system and disrupt the body's delicate chemical and electrical balance. The end result is mental and physical disease.

The stress reaction is a primitive response to a threatening or dangerous situation. It is commonly referred to as the 'fight-or-flight' syndrome. When confronted with a situation we perceive as threatening, the sympathetic nervous system activates involuntary responses designed to activate all the major systems of the body.

When the body prepares for 'fight-or-flight', it does so with short-term goals in mind. Fuel is released in the form of glucose or stored blood sugar. More blood is sent to the muscles. Air passages relax and a sense of stimulation is produced. The adrenal glands release adrenaline and noradrenaline into the blood stream. These two hormones mimic the actions of nervous stimulation in a number of organs in the body. The heart rate increases, blood vessels dilate in some areas and constrict in others, the rate of respiration increases and most digestive activities slow down or stop altogether. Digestion and excretion are not high priorities, so adrenaline causes vascular constriction which reduces the flow of blood to these areas. By all this we are prepared for a short burst of heightened activity.

In modern society many influences can trigger this response. Most of these cannot be handled with a short burst of activity. So the body's response is repressed. Often stress situations are continuous, so stress responses are semi-permanently on red alert – a situation which cannot be maintained for too long without the body suffering from extreme exhaustion. The stress build-up eventually explodes internally and knocks our systems out of balance.

Long-term adrenal stimulation with no discharge of energy will deplete essential minerals and vitamins from the system, for example Vitamins B and C, which are vital to the functioning of the immune system. This will result in lowered resistance and increased susceptibility to diseases directly related to a lowered immune system – such as ME and AIDS. Long-term adrenal build-up can also affect blood pressure and cause a build-up of fatty substances on blood vessel walls, as well as damage the functioning of the digestive system.

Stress affects different people in different ways and to varying degrees. One person may exhibit cardiovascular problems, another gastrointestinal upset, anorexia, palpitations, sweating or headaches – to mention but a few of the myriad of bodily reactions to stress. The cardiovascular and digestive systems are obvious candidates for the ill-effects of stress – high blood pressure, ulcers, indigestion and the like. Stress can also be linked to infectious diseases. When the body is busy with the effects of residual stress, it cannot organize an effective defence against invading organisms. It is a vicious cycle.

Reflexology helps alleviate the effects of stress by inducing deep relaxation, and thereby allowing the nervous system to function normally and free the body to seek its own homoeostasis. Tension is relaxed, vascular constriction reduced and blood and nerve supply flow more freely, allowing oxygen and nutrients to make their way to where they are needed. Reflexology is a powerful antidote to stress. A relaxed balanced body can heal itself and reflexology is a guaranteed method of relaxing the body and balancing the biological systems.

Reflexology Improves Circulation

One of Eunice Ingham's favourite sayings was 'Circulation is life. Stagnation is death.' Every practitioner acknowledges the importance of good circulation. If the smallest fraction of circulation is cut off from one or more parts of the body, the effects soon become evident as a variety of aches and pains.

Blood carries oxygen and nutrients to the cells and removes waste products and toxins from the cells. During this process blood vessels contract and relax so their resilience is most important for proper functioning. Stress and tension tighten up the cardiovascular system and restrict blood flow. Circulation becomes sluggish, causing high or low blood pressure.

High blood pressure can cause numerous problems – for example arteriosclerosis or hardening of the arteries. The increased pressure forces materials into the walls of the arteries. These materials build up, coating the insides. Blood flow is reduced, which signals a hormone in the kidneys to be released and the pressure is further increased. The heart, brain and kidneys could be affected.

Reduced blood flow to the organs inhibits the oxygen supply and nutrients to the cells. Without oxygen, cells die. Without the proper nutrients, cells fail to function efficiently. The glands and organs begin to malfunction and lose their balancing qualities; this could cause them to overreact or underreact.

A good example of the body's balancing act is the pancreas. One of its jobs is to maintain the balance of glucose, or blood sugar. This is achieved with the hormone insulin, which activates the body cells to take up the glucose from the blood. Without insulin, the glucose is not consumed or is stored improperly. It accumulates in the blood, causing the dangerous condition diabetes. If there is an excess of insulin produced, the opposite effect occurs. When insulin removes glucose from the blood, the storage of glucose in the form of glycogen is increased at the expense of the blood. Low blood sugar/hypoglycaemia is the result. The balancing act has been upset. Glands and organs depend on equilibrium, and on the blood circulation to bring the needed elements.

With improved circulation, the body is cleansed of toxins and impurities. If the body's built-in cleansing systems – the lymphatic and excretory systems – become blocked or function improperly, toxins and waste matter build up. The increased state of relaxation facilitated by reflexology allows the body systems – including the excretory systems – to function efficiently and waste is properly eliminated. By reducing stress and tension, reflexology allows the cardiovascular vessels to conduct the flow of blood naturally and easily.

Reflexology Improves Nerve Function

The organs and glands contribute to the overall well-being of the body – each making contributions to maintaining an efficient, fully operated mechanism. But all receive their instructions from the most intricate of all networks, the nerves. These cord-like structures, comprised of a collection of nerve fibres, convey impulses between a part of the central nervous system and other regions of the body. Problems can often be caused by tension putting pressure on a vital nerve plexus or even a single nerve structure supplying a vital organ. As tension is eased, pressure on the nerves and vessels is relaxed, thus improving the flow of blood and its supply of oxygen and nutrients to all parts of the body.

Every part of the body is operated by messages carried back and forth along neural pathways. Stimulation of sensory nerve endings sends information to the spinal cord and brain. The brain and spinal cord send instructions to the organs and muscles. The neural pathways are both living tissue and electrical channels and can be impinged upon or polluted by many factors. When neural pathways are impaired nerve function is impeded – messages are delivered slowly and unreliably, or not at all, and body processes operate at less than optimum levels. Reflexology, by stimulating the thousands of nerve endings in the feet, encourages the opening and clearing of neural pathways.

Reflexology Revitalizes Energy and Rebalances the Whole System

The body is a dynamic energy field; energy circulates throughout the body. For optimum functioning, energy must flow unimpeded and the yin and yang energy currents must complement each other. Reflexology opens up these energy pathways, energizing the physical, emotional and mental aspects of the body. When the body is 'out of balance', it is not functioning efficiently. We are all easily thrown off balance by stress, attitudes, lifestyle and diet. Reflexology helps return the body to a dynamic state of balance.

WHO CAN BENEFIT FROM REFLEXOLOGY?

Reflexology doesn't discriminate. There are no boundaries or limitations. People of any race, age, colour or creed, men, women, teenagers, children, babies and the elderly – all can enjoy the positive benefits reflexology has to offer. As reflexology can do no harm, the only restrictions are those determined by the clients' pain threshold and their reactions to massage. Elderly people with no specific complaint will benefit from a couple of courses of treatment a year to keep the bodily functions toned and for a sense of well-being. Results are also good with children and babies because they are more relaxed and supple and because their bodies are highly receptive to therapeutic stimuli.

Reflexologists Don't . . .

Reflexologists don't practise medicine. According to the law, only licensed physicians are allowed to do that. Reflexologists *never* diagnose a disease, treat for a specific condition, prescribe or adjust medication. They do not treat specific diseases although they help eliminate problems caused by specific diseases. By bringing the body back into a state of balance, treatment can combat a number of disorders. Tender reflexes indicate which parts of the body are congested. This 'diagnosis' is only of parts of the body 'out of balance' and not specific, named disorders.

The Reflexology Treatment

A reflexology treatment should always be a most pleasant experience. A client may be tense and apprehensive on the first visit, but any good practitioner will always make an effort to relax the client and give full, undivided attention. The practitioner will require a thorough medical history in as much detail as possible, as all problems, not only those specifically causing trouble at the time, are relevant in ascertaining a complete health picture of the client.

Many people are embarrassed about their feet. When visiting a reflexologist, any insecurity regarding the state of your feet should be forgotten. To a reflexologist, your feet represent your body and they tell a thousand stories about the state of the body. Every nick and crevice holds a key to the nature of the problem. And reflexology is the key to relieving these.

Comfort is the first prerequisite in the treatment so correct positioning is important. The client will be seated comfortably, preferably on a soft treatment couch with the head and upper part of the body upright – the head and neck well supported, so the client and reflexologist have eye contact. The lower legs will be well supported with the feet in a comfortable position. Shoes and stockings must be removed and tight garments should be loosened so as not to hinder circulation.

The practitioner begins by disinfecting the feet and the first physical contact is usually a gentle stroking movement, before the practitioner proceeds with a general examination of the feet. As every individual is different, so too are their feet, which reveal a variety of characteristics peculiar to that particular person.

Temperature, static build-up, muscle tone and tissue tone and skin condition are all noted as the therapist tries to get as comprehensive a view of the client as possible. Cold, bluish or reddish feet indicate poor circulation. Feet that perspire indicate a glandular imbalance. Dry skin could indicate poor circulation. Callouses, corns, bunions and the like, and their possible links, will also be noted. (Further information on this in Chapter 3.) Care must be taken with infectious areas as they could spread to other areas of the foot and to the practitioner. These should be covered with a plaster or cotton wool before they are worked on. Working on varicose veins should be avoided as it could further damage the veins. Swelling and puffiness, especially around the ankles, can relate to internal problems. Tense feet may indicate tension in the body, and limp feet may indicate poor muscle tone.

What the Reflexology Treatment Feels Like

In one word – wonderful. Calming, comforting and exhilarating. It is certainly not ticklish, since the massage technique is too firm to tickle. The foot massage technique is different to other forms of massage. The thumb is the most important working 'tool' used to apply pressure to the reflex areas – each of which is about the size of a pinhead. The foot is always well supported and the pressure firm but not agonizing.

Sensations vary on different parts of the feet, depending on the functioning of the related body parts. Congested areas will be sensitive – the more sensitive it is, the more congested it is. The sensations range from the feeling of something sharp (like a piece of glass) being pressed into the foot to a dull ache, discomfort, tightness or just firm pressure. Sensitivity varies from person to person. For example, some people may be relatively unhealthy and have insensitive reflexes, while others may be reasonably healthy and have tender reflexes. This also varies from treatment to treatment, depending on factors such as stress, mood and time of day. In many cases, a client may feel little or no tenderness at all during the first treatment. This does not necessarily mean no areas are congested. It more often than not indicates an energy blockage in the feet which needs to be freed. The feet usually become more sensitive with subsequent treatments.

As treatment progresses, tenderness should diminish. The treatment should never be painful or cause the client any discomfort. The practitioner will adjust pressure to suit the client. No matter what the sensations, treatment is always effective and should leave the client feeling light, tingly and thoroughly pampered.

Reactions to Reflexology Treatment

People differ, so do reactions. On the whole, reactions immediately after a reflexology treatment are largely pleasant – calm and relaxed or energized and rejuvenated. However, there is some bad with the good. Reflexology activates the body's healing power, so some form of reaction is inevitable as the body rids itself of toxins. This is referred to as a 'healing crisis' and is usually a cleansing process. The severity of reactions depends on the degree of imbalance, but should never be too radical. The most common phrase following a first treatment is 'I have never slept so well!'

Most common reactions are cleansing reactions which manifest in the eliminating systems of the body – the kidneys, bowels, skin and lungs. The following reactions are not unusual:

– increased urination as the kidneys are stimulated to produce more urine, which may also be darker and stronger smelling due to the toxic content
– flatulence and more frequent bowel movements
– aggravated skin conditions, particularly those that have been suppressed; increased perspiration and pimples
– improved skin tone and tissue texture due to improved circulation
– increased secretions of the mucous membranes in the nose, mouth and bronchi
– disrupted sleep patterns – either deeper or more disturbed sleep
– dizziness or nausea
– a temporary outbreak of a disease which has been suppressed
– increased discharge from the vagina in women
– feverishness
– tiredness

Whatever the reactions, however, they are a necessary part of the healing process and will pass. It is a good idea to drink a lot of water (preferably boiled) to help flush the toxins out as fast as possible.

Length of a Reflexology Treatment

The length of treatment and number of sessions will vary depending on the client and the condition – for example, the patient's constitution, the history and nature of his illness, his age, the ability of his body to react to the treatments, his way of life and his attitude to the treatment.

The first treatment is investigative and exploratory and should take about an hour. Following treatments would be thirty to forty minutes. If the session is too short, insufficient stimulus is provided for the body to mobilize its own healing powers; if it is too long, there is a danger of overstimulating which can cause excessive elimination and discomfort.

An effect is often experienced immediately after the first treatment. Generally results are apparent after three to four treatments – either complete or considerable improvement. Disorders present for a long time take longer to correct than those present for a short time. A course of treatments is recommended for all conditions (even if one session appears to have corrected the problem) to balance the body totally and prevent a recurrence of the disorder. The course should be eight to twelve treatments once or twice a week. For optimum results two sessions a week are recommended until there is an improvement, then the frequency can gradually be reduced.

If there is no reaction after several sessions, the body could be unreceptive, due to external factors, such as heavy medication or psychological attitude, which are blocking the therapeutic impulses. As long as reactions are positive there is value in continuing the treatment.

In cases of severe illness such as cancer, multiple sclerosis or paralysis, reflexology may not remove the cause of the disease, but it can significantly improve the patient's general condition as it helps relieve pain; activates the excretory organs; stimulates the respiratory system and helps the patient achieve better control of bladder and bowels.

PREVENTATIVE THERAPY

Health-threatening dangers lurk around every corner of our modern environment: polluted land, air and water, contaminated and irradiated food, a completely contaminated environment. Add to this the stress of our day-to-day lives – bad diet, attitudes and lifestyle – and we have a potentially lethal cocktail designed to attract disease. Most people wait until disease rears its ugly head before they seek help. But it makes far more sense to listen to the body's warning signals and take action early. Apart from caring for the body by eating more sensibly, exercising and calming the mind and body through relaxation and meditation techniques, occasional visits to a reflexologist as extra 'maintenance' can be of enormous benefit to all.

Preventative therapy is useful for people who have completed a course of treatment and want to continue it to avoid any problems re-emerging, as well as for those who may not have any acute symptoms but realize the need for preventative action. Treatments at regular intervals can assist the body in maintaining a balanced state, and prevent the possibility of slight imbalances from becoming troublesome. It is possible to detect imbalances in the early stages and prevent more serious problems occurring. The intervals between treatments will vary from person to person and may involve weeks or months. For best results, treatment should be applied in the correct manner by a trained therapist, but it can also be beneficial for clients to work on certain reflexes themselves between sessions, to act as a boost to the treatment. To quote Avi Grinberg in *Holistic Reflexology*:

The truly successful treatment is not the one that saves the person from a condition that is in its advanced stage, but is one that prevents its development into a serious or chronic condition.

Healing is always a possibility. There are many components of healing beyond the physical. So with reflexology, even though we may be working on the physical level, we still need to be quite conscious of the mental, emotional and spiritual levels. Healing usually occurs when these three elements are recognized. There needs to be a balance between the body and its environment, the physical, emotional and mental conditions. Clients need to be in balance with the individuals and relationships in their lives – relationships at school, work, or during leisure time. All these things need to be balanced and then healing can occur.

Rest, a change of environment, or most importantly, a change in attitude can allow this balance to be restored. Often we do not get the rest we would like, or cannot change our environment, but a change in attitude can have astounding benefits.

This change in attitude is very important. Many people feel the need to talk during a session. By talking about what is happening in their lives, they can sometimes come to a new understanding of their problems. Or perhaps the reflexologist can suggest a different perspective or approach to a problem in a non-judgmental way. This helps the client relax and see that a change in attitude is possible. This new attitude may allow clients to make changes in their environment and this in turn will help the body to function in a state of balance or homoeostasis – the major goal of reflexology.

3

Meridians

MERIDIANS AND REFLEXOLOGY

The concept of energy channels is the central point around which the practices of reflexology and acupuncture are based. Both are based on the premise that vital energy is channelled along various lines throughout the body. In acupuncture, the lines are known as meridians; in reflexology, zones. Both ascertain that disease is caused by blockages in energy lines, and treatment involves clearing out these obstructions by stimulating various points along the lines. In acupuncture, points situated all over the body are stimulated by needles. Reflexology concentrates only on reflex areas and sections of meridians found on the feet which are stimulated by a specific massage technique.

The similarity between the two therapies seems to be more than just coincidence. When Dr Fitzgerald developed the zone theory in the early 1900s, the Chinese concept of meridians was completely unknown in the West. Fitzgerald's 'discovery' of the existence of energy lines was undoubtedly a breakthrough and an invaluable contribution to the re-emergence of reflexology in the West. But it seems very likely and also a logical assumption that the energy lines Fitzgerald stumbled upon were, in fact, the meridians understood by the Chinese for thousands of years.

Closer study of the meridians reveals that the six main meridians are found in the feet, specifically the toes. Thus, massaging the feet is, in actual fact, stimulating and clearing congestions in the meridians. When congestions are cleared, energy is able to flow freely and the body is able to achieve a state of balance.

The six main meridians are those which actually penetrate the major body organs – the liver, spleen/pancreas, stomach, gall bladder, bladder and kidney. The other six meridians – lung, large intestine, pericardium/circulation, Three E/endocrine, small intestine and heart – are situated in the arms and do not actually penetrate specific organs. However, as the meridian cycle is one continuous energy flow, the six meridians which do not penetrate organs are indirectly stimulated when the main meridians are worked on. This is due to the fact that the organs related to these meridians are found along the six main meridians. For example, the lung meridian runs along the arm down to the thumb, but the lung itself is penetrated by the stomach meridian, and therefore congestions would be indirectly affected by stimulating the stomach meridian.

Meridians have a long and authentic history. The Chinese discovered the meridian system approximately 3000 years ago. The fact that this system has been used successfully all this time, and is going from strength to strength, particularly in the West, is proof of its efficacy. It is a logical progression to now incorporate meridians into the realm of reflexology in order to advance and enhance this holistic health therapy.

An understanding of meridians can help reflexologists to understand the disease pathway more comprehensively. A basic knowledge of meridians can be of enormous benefit in pinpointing problems. If, for example, pain, irritation or any other condition does not improve satisfactorily through treatment of the reflex area, one should observe the meridian which traverses the part of the body in question, and treat the reflex area of the organ related to that meridian. The meridians can be used simply and effectively for a better understanding of conditions. For example, a client has arthritis in the little finger, tennis elbow, fibrositis in the shoulder muscles, infection in the lymph glands of the throat, trigeminal neuralgia and hearing diseases. One need simply look at the small intestine meridian which starts in the little finger and ends just in front of the ear and passes the locations of all the above disorders. Could this mean that the small intestine disorder could aggravate or even cause these problems? Clinical results of balancing the meridians certainly indicate this.

WHAT ARE MERIDIANS?

All life and matter is energy operating at various frequencies. This energy, known as ch'i or life-force, is what keeps us alive. The Chinese discovered that this ch'i circulates in the body along 'meridians', similar to the blood, nerve and lymphatic circuits. This vital life-force controls the workings of the main organs and systems of the body. It circulates from one organ to another. For each organ to maintain a perfect state of health, the ch'i energy must be able to flow freely along the meridians. If this is balanced, it is impossible to be ill in body, mind or spirit. All illness is a result of an imbalance in the energy flow.

Meridians are located throughout the body. They have been described as containing a free-flowing, colourless, non-cellular liquid which may be partly actuated by the heart (*Handbook of Acupressure II*, by Iona Marsaa-Teergurden). Meridians have been measured and mapped by modern technological methods, electronically, thermatically and radioactively. With practice they can be felt. There are specific acupuncture points along the meridians. These points are electromagnetic in character and consist of small oval cells called Bonham Corpuscles which surround the capillaries in the skin, the blood vessels and the organs throughout the body. There are some five hundred points which are most frequently used. They are stimulated in a definite sequence depending on the action required. Meridians are named by the live functions with which they seem to associate. In most cases, this name is the same as that of many of the gross organs we are familiar with.

The Chinese maintain that the ch'i circulates in the meridians twenty-five times a day and twenty-five times a night. In a sense, there is only one single meridian which goes right round the entire body, but many different meridians are described according to their positions and functions. There are twelve main meridians which are bilateral (paired) resulting in twenty-four separate pathways. Each meridian is connected and related to a specific organ from which it gets its name. It is also connected to a partner meridian and organ with which it has a specific relationship. The partner meridians each consist of a yin and a yang meridian/organ and come under the dominance of one of the five elements.

The twelve main meridians control the lungs, large intestine, stomach, spleen/pancreas, heart, small intestine, bladder, kidney, pericardium, 'triple warmer', gall-bladder and liver. Within our bodies the yang organs are those which are hollow and involved in absorption and discharge such as the stomach and bladder; the yin organs are the dense, blood-filled organs such as the heart, which regulate the body. There is constant interaction between yin and yang forces and, if the yin/yang balance between the organs is interrupted, the flow of ch'i throughout the body will be affected and we will fall ill.

The acupuncturist balances this ch'i with needles, and sometimes laser equipment. In shiatsu, the same effect is achieved utilizing finger pressure. In the VacuFlex Reflexology System (described later in the book) rubber cups are used. These cups which suction on to the body are strategically placed on a particular meridian and thereby balance the energy flow.

The Meridian Cycle

Meridians are classified yin or yang on the basis of the direction in which they flow on the surface of the body. Meridians interconnect deep within the torso and have an internal branch and a surface branch. The section worked on is the surface branch which is accessible to touch techniques. Yang energy flows from the sun and yang meridians run from the fingers to the face, or from the face to the feet. Yin energy from the earth flows from the feet to the torso and from the torso along the inside (yin side) of the arms to the fingertips. Since the meridian flow is actually one long continuous unbroken flow, the energy flows in one definite direction and from one meridian to another in a well-determined order. Because there is no beginning or end to this flow, the order of the meridian is represented as a wheel. As we go round this wheel following the meridian line, the flow follows this order of the body:

– from torso to fingertips – along the inside of the arm = yin.
– from fingertips to face – along the outside/back of the arm = yang.
– from face to feet – along the outside of the leg = yang.
– from feet to torso – along the inside of the leg = yin.

The Chinese Clock/Midday-Midnight Law

The Chinese recognized a twenty-four hour movement of energy referred to as the Chinese Clock. This 'clock' is a twenty-four hour cycle which divides the day and night into two-hour periods. Each one of these is associated with a surge of energy in one of the organs and its meridian. For example, between the hours of 3 and 5 am, the lungs receive their daily booster. The cycle begins with the lungs and for this reason it is said that these are the hours when it is most suitable to be born.

The Chinese believe that the best time for stimulating a particular organ is at the two-hour period when its energy is 'full'. Alternatively, it should be sedated at the opposite period of the day or night. For example the lungs should be stimulated between 3 and 5 am and sedated between 3 and 5 pm. The opposite treatment should be applied at the opposite time on the clock. The organ maximum energy periods are included in the detailed section on meridians.

The Five Elements

Meridian therapy and acupuncture can be more clearly understood in the light of the Chinese belief that five elements comprise the world, and that everything on earth essentially falls into the category of one or more of these elements.

The five elements are generated and destroyed according to a law of cyclical interaction: fire produces earth, earth produces metal, metal finds water, water produces wood and wood becomes fire. By substituting for each element a corresponding yin organ, for example, we see that the heart (fire) aids or reinforces the action of the spleen/pancreas (earth); the spleen/pancreas the lungs (metal); the lungs the kidneys (water); the kidneys the liver (wood) and the liver the heart.

Conversely, just as fire melts metal, metal cuts down wood, wood covers earth, earth absorbs water and water puts out fire, so the diseased or malfunctioning heart adversely affects the action of the lungs, the lungs affect the liver, the liver affects the spleen/pancreas, and the spleen/pancreas affects the kidneys and the kidneys affect the heart. So, to the Chinese, the nourishing and inhibiting cycle relates not only to the construction and working of the universe, but to the human body as well.

From another aspect, the mind fuels the body with negative or positive thoughts. Negative thoughts breed destructive elements. Destructive elements create tension and constrictions of circulation. Disease manifests in tense, sluggish areas of the body. The organs become diseased and fail to function. Our thinking becomes even more disturbed and negative. Pain permeates most of our days which causes us to become more and more dissociated from nature. Our vital energy becomes weaker and weaker until eventually we die and go back to the earth.

Each of the five elements is assigned at least one yin and one yang organ. They are identified with the five elements in the following manner:

Fire: yin – heart, pericardium (circulation)
 yang – small intestine, triple warmer
Earth: yin – spleen/pancreas
 yang – stomach
Metal: yin – lungs
 yang – large intestine
Water: yin – kidneys
 yang – bladder
Wood: yin – liver
 yang – gall bladder

Symptoms/Signs to Note Along Meridians

Before we look into the meridians and their symptoms, we will take a brief look at the disorders and congestions which can occur along the meridians and indicate where problems may lie. These may take the form of skin disorders, warts, birthmarks, lumps, nail problems and the like.

If a person has skin problems, it may be obvious that the lung and large intestine are the root cause, but note must be taken of exactly where the problem manifests on the body; down the legs, for example, or on the back. Often these will occur parallel to each other. For example, someone with psoriasis may have it on the outer side of the leg (gall bladder meridian) and down the back (bladder meridian).

Look at the nails for white spots, ridges, problems with the root of the nails or any other nail defects. Ridges often indicate high acidity, and if you take note on which meridian it manifests, you will see where the congestion occurs – for example, if it is on the thumb, the acidity is congesting the lung meridian. If there are white spots on the nails, these indicate a deficiency. As the nail takes approximately three months to grow, divide the nail into segments. The centre, for example, indicates approximately six weeks. One can thereby ascertain the approximate period when the deficiency occurred and relate it to the situation at the time – for example, the person may have been on a sugar binge or through a great deal of stress which caused the deficiency. Always note these signs, and pinpoint the meridian on which they appear in order to trace the problem organ.

MERIDIANS

Lung Meridian
Yin meridian
Partner meridian – Large Intestine – Yang
Element – Metal
Organ Maximum Energy Period – 3 am to 5 am

The lungs and large intestine control elimination; the former carbon dioxide, the latter solid residue. As these meridians are

31

partnered, they can directly affect each other – for example chest problems can be accompanied by constipation and vice versa.

The lungs regulate respiration. They are responsible for taking ch'i from the air and for regulating the states of ch'i in the body. Healthy lungs and regular even respiration ensure that ch'i enters and leaves the body smoothly. An imbalance results in symptoms such as asthma, coughs and various forms of chest congestion. Respiratory functions affect all the rhythms of the body including the blood flow.

The lungs are called the 'tender' organ because they are the most easily influenced by environmental factors and are involved with regulating sweat secretion which increases resistance to external environmental influences.

Large Intestine Meridian
Yang meridian
Partner Meridian – Lung – Yin
Element – Metal
Organ Maximum Energy Period – 5 am to 7 am

'The large intestine forms the lower part of the digestive tract and is in charge of transporting, transforming and eliminating surplus matter. If these wastes are not eliminated regularly, it can have a toxic effect on the entire system. Thus *mental* constipation – toxic thoughts and feelings – are often associated with this meridian, in addition to *physical* constipation or diarrhoea,' to quote from Iona Marsaa-Teegurden's '*Acupressure Handbook*'.

The *Nei Ching* refers to the large intestine as the generator of evolution and change – and as being integral to the well-being of the whole body. The important function of elimination of waste material is vital to the maintenance of health. If waste is not effectively excreted, the rest of the system has to cope with an additional load of toxic waste and this will cause disharmony throughout the body. An imbalance in the large intestine can result in abdominal pain, diarrhoea, constipation, bloatedness, swelling, acne and boils, headaches and stuffy nose.

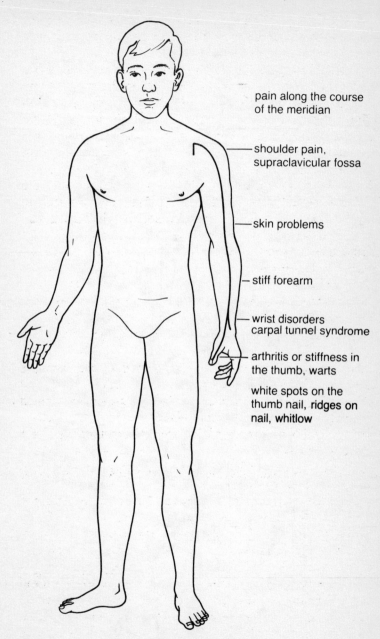

pain along the course
of the meridian

shoulder pain,
supraclavicular fossa

skin problems

stiff forearm

wrist disorders
carpal tunnel syndrome

arthritis or stiffness in
the thumb, warts

white spots on the
thumb nail, **ridges on
nail, whitlow**

Fig. 3. The lung meridian

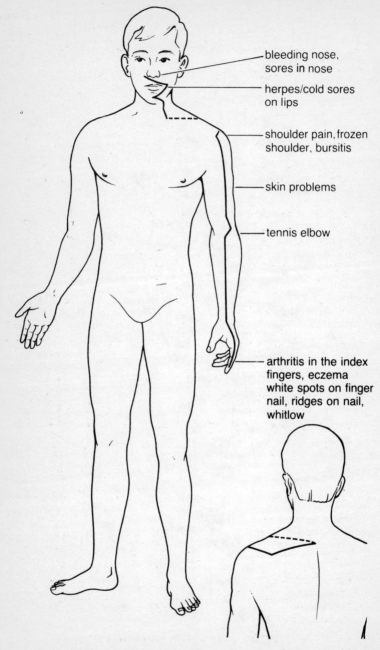

Fig. 4. *The large intestine (colon) meridian*

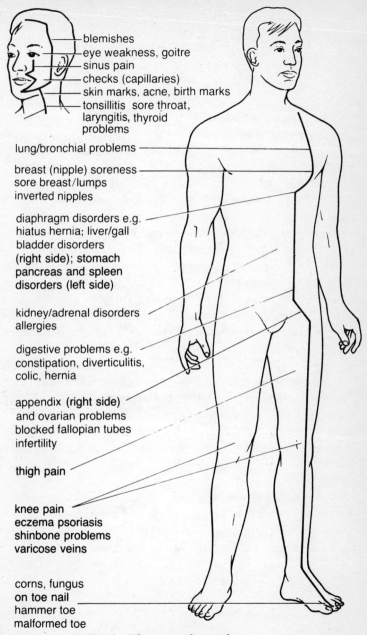

blemishes
eye weakness, goitre
sinus pain
checks (capillaries)
skin marks, acne, birth marks
tonsillitis sore throat,
laryngitis, thyroid
problems

lung/bronchial problems

breast (nipple) soreness
sore breast/lumps
inverted nipples

diaphragm disorders e.g.
hiatus hernia; liver/gall
bladder disorders
(right side); stomach
pancreas and spleen
disorders (left side)

kidney/adrenal disorders
allergies

digestive problems e.g.
constipation, diverticulitis,
colic, hernia

appendix (right side)
and ovarian problems
blocked fallopian tubes
infertility

thigh pain

knee pain
eczema psoriasis
shinbone problems
varicose veins

corns, fungus
on toe nail
hammer toe
malformed toe

Fig.5. The stomach meridian

Stomach Meridian
Yang Meridian
Partner Meridian – Spleen/Pancreas – Yin
Element – Earth
Organ Maximum Energy Period – 7 am to 9 am

The functions and activities of the stomach and spleen are closely related. The stomach controls digestion – it receives nourishment, integrates it and passes on the 'pure' food energy to be distributed by the spleen. The spleen then transforms it into the raw material for ch'i and blood. If the stomach does not hold and digest food, the spleen cannot transform it and transport its essence. They are interdependent meridians.

According to Chinese philosophy, the stomach is related to appetite, digestion and transport of food and liquid, but the ruler of food transport and energy consumption is the stomach's partner, the spleen/pancreas.

The two meridians of the earth element work together more closely than any of the others to stabilize the individual. The earth element represents harmony and if there is no harmony in the stomach, pancreas and spleen, this will affect all the other organs.

The stomach is referred to by the Chinese as the 'sea of food and fluid' as it governs digestion and is responsible for 'receiving' and 'ripening' ingested food and fluids. Without the nourishing activities of the stomach the other organs in the body could not function. The stomach is *central* physically and functionally; thus, according to Oriental therapists *any problem in the stomach is quickly reflected in the other organs*.

If this organ is out of balance, whatever is taken in, be it physical or psychic food, will not be utilized correctly. Energy depletion – lethargy, weakness and debilitation are symptoms warning us that the function of this organ is impaired.

Spleen/Pancreas Meridian
Yin Meridian
Partner Meridian – Stomach – Yang
Element – Earth
Organ Maximum Energy Period – 9 am to 11 am

A traditional saying that combines the meaning of several references in the *Nei Ching* states that 'the spleen rules transformation and transportation'. It is the crucial link in the process by which food is transformed into ch'i and blood. If this process of food transformation is not activated nourishment and ch'i are not available for the muscles so they become weak and the lips and mouth become pale and dry. The spleen is traditionally referred to as the 'foundation of postnatal existence'. If the spleen is imbalanced the whole body or some part of it may develop deficient ch'i or deficient blood.

Physiologically, the pancreas has considerable control over the body's nourishment, since its secretions help digest all the main kinds of food: proteins, fats and starch.

According to the Chinese, 'The spleen governs the blood'; it helps create blood and keeps it flowing in its proper paths. It therefore also influences menstruation. The spleen destroys spent red blood cells and forms antibodies which neutralize poisonous bacteria, thus influencing immunity to infection. Another important function of this meridian has to do with the transformation of liquids; the classics say that oedema (swelling from retention of excess fluids) is related to the spleen.

Heart Meridian
Yin Meridian
Partner Meridian – Small Intestine – Yang
Element – Fire
Organ Maximum Energy Period – 11 am to 1 pm

The heart and small intestine meridians are coupled; the *Nei Ching* explains their relationship: 'The heart controls the blood and unites with the small intestine. If the heart becomes heated, the heat will converge in the small intestine, producing blood in the urine.'

The classics say, 'The heart rules the blood and blood vessels.' It regulates the blood flow, so when the heart is functioning properly, the blood flows smoothly. If the heart is strong, the body will be healthy and the emotions orderly; if it is weak, all the other meridians will be disturbed.

It is also said that the heart rules the spirit. So, when the heart's blood and ch'i are harmonious, spirit is nourished and

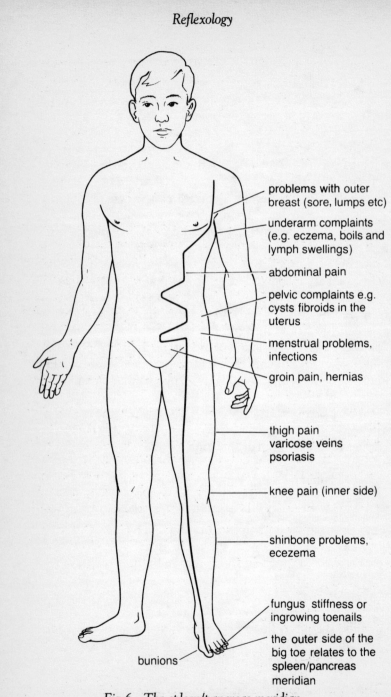

problems with outer breast (sore, lumps etc)

underarm complaints (e.g. eczema, boils and lymph swellings)

abdominal pain

pelvic complaints e.g. cysts fibroids in the uterus

menstrual problems, infections

groin pain, hernias

thigh pain varicose veins psoriasis

knee pain (inner side)

shinbone problems, ecezema

fungus stiffness or ingrowing toenails

the outer side of the big toe relates to the spleen/pancreas meridian

bunions

Fig. 6. The spleen/pancreas meridian

the individual responds appropriately to the environment. If this is impaired symptoms like insomnia, excessive dreaming, forgetfulness, hysteria, irrational behaviour, insanity and delirium may manifest.

Small Intestine Meridian
Yang Meridian
Partner Meridian – Heart – Yin
Element – Fire
Organ Maximum Energy Period – 1 pm to 3 pm

The small intestine meridian rules the separation of the 'pure' and the 'impure'. It continues the process of separation and absorption of food begun in the stomach. Because the meridian is in charge of assimilation this flow has considerable influence over body nourishment and body-mind vitality.

The small intestine influences the functioning of the large intestine both directly and indirectly. In addition to passing solid residue on to the large intestine, the small intestine also controls the proportion of liquid to solid matter in the faeces, reabsorbing some liquids for the body's use and passing some on to be eliminated.

The 'sorting out' process – keeping that which has value and passing on waste to where it can be removed – happens on all levels, both physiological and psychological, for example in sorting out the 'rubbish' from that which is useful in terms of ideas, emotions and thoughts. If this function is not operating efficiently symptoms that express this confusion may arise – for example hearing difficulties, such as the inability to distinguish different sounds. Thus the flow relates not only to assimilation of foodstuffs but also to assimilation of experience, feelings and ideas and to spiritual nourishment.

Bladder Meridian
Yang Meridian
Partner Meridian – Kidney – Yin
Element – Water
Organ Maximum Energy Period – 3 pm to 5 pm

The partnership of the kidney and bladder meridians is one of

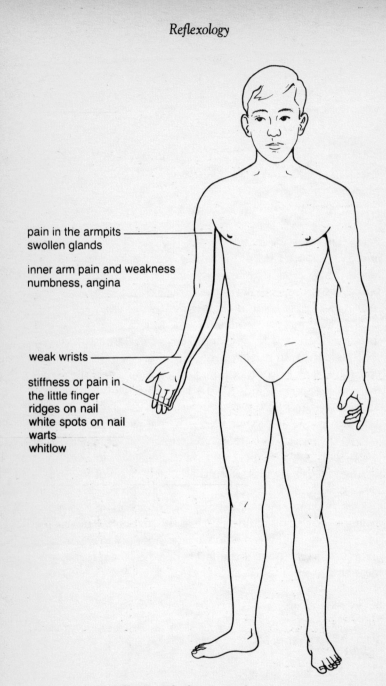

pain in the armpits
swollen glands

inner arm pain and weakness
numbness, angina

weak wrists

stiffness or pain in
the little finger
ridges on nail
white spots on nail
warts
whitlow

Fig. 7. The heart meridian

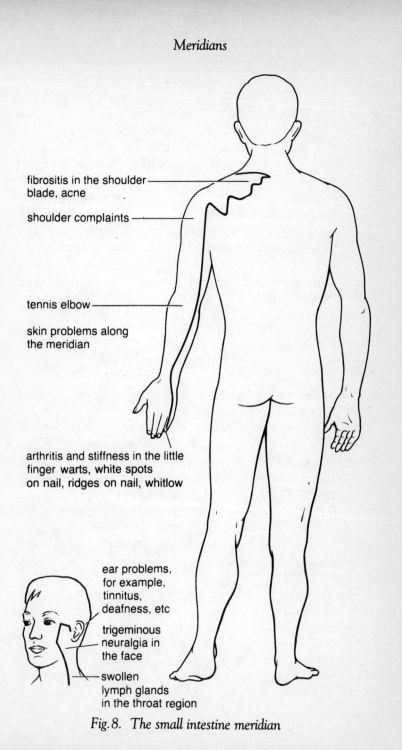

fibrositis in the shoulder blade, acne

shoulder complaints

tennis elbow

skin problems along the meridian

arthritis and stiffness in the little finger warts, white spots on nail, ridges on nail, whitlow

ear problems, for example, tinnitus, deafness, etc

trigeminous neuralgia in the face

swollen lymph glands in the throat region

Fig.8. The small intestine meridian

the most obvious and means that the bladder meridian has a role in stimulating and regulating the kidneys.

The function of the bladder is to receive and excrete urine produced in the kidneys, and the meridian is therefore in charge of maintaining normal fluid levels in the body. It is also coupled with the function of the kidney in helping to store the vital essence (see below). The bladder is essential to life because if it is not functioning, the rest of the system becomes poisoned and stressed beyond endurance.

The bladder meridian strongly affects the spinal cord and nerves and it is most effective to release the tensions along its route.

Kidney Meridian
Yin Meridian
Partner Meridian – Bladder – Yang
Element – Water
Organ Maximum Energy Period – 5 pm to 7 pm

The *Nei Ching* states: 'When the kidneys are deficient . . . the spirit becomes easily provoked.'

'The kidneys store the Jing' and rule birth, development and maturation. Jing is the substance – a vital essence – that is the source of life and individual development. It has the potential for differentiation into yin and yang and therefore produces life. The body and all the organs need Jing to thrive, and because the kidneys store Jing, they bestow this potential for life activity. They have therefore a special relationship with the other organs because the yin and yang, or life activity of each organ ultimately depends on the yin and yang of the kidneys.

The kidneys regulate the amount of water in the body. Fluid is essential to life. The flow of the fluid enables waste material to be collected and excreted in the form of urine. Enormous amounts of blood flow through the kidneys to be purified. If the blood does not flow as it should symptoms such as high blood pressure or hypertension may result and there may be a build-up of toxic substances that the body would be unable to deal with.

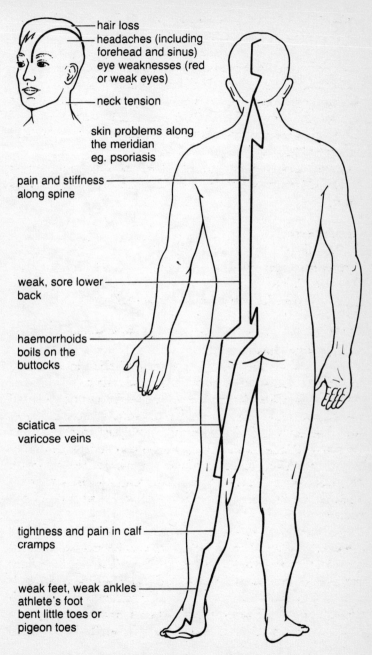

hair loss

headaches (including forehead and sinus)
eye weaknesses (red or weak eyes)

neck tension

skin problems along the meridian eg. psoriasis

pain and stiffness along spine

weak, sore lower back

haemorrhoids boils on the buttocks

sciatica varicose veins

tightness and pain in calf cramps

weak feet, weak ankles athlete's foot bent little toes or pigeon toes

Fig. 9. The bladder meridian

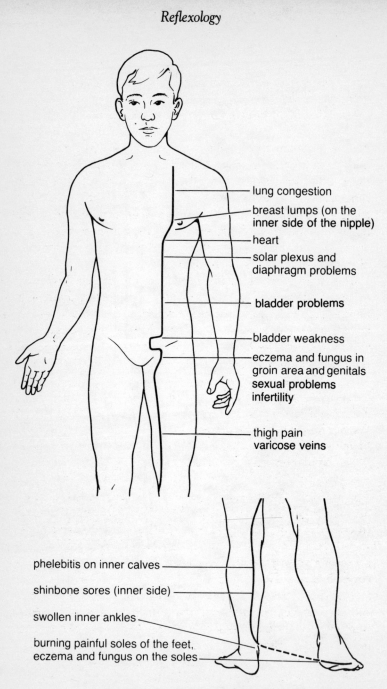

lung congestion

breast lumps (on the inner side of the nipple)

heart

solar plexus and diaphragm problems

bladder problems

bladder weakness

eczema and fungus in groin area and genitals
sexual problems
infertility

thigh pain
varicose veins

phelebitis on inner calves

shinbone sores (inner side)

swollen inner ankles

burning painful soles of the feet, eczema and fungus on the soles

Fig. 10. The kidney meridian

Circulation/Pericardium Meridian
Yin Meridian
Partner Meridian – Endocrine/Triple Warmer/ Three E – Yang
Element – Fire
Organ Maximum Energy Period – 7 pm to 9 pm

The pericardium and triple warmer are coupled meridians and both have protective functions. The pericardium protects the heart – the ruler – and the triple warmer protects the other nine meridians. The condition of either affects the other; if the triple warmer is imbalanced, the organs are deprived of proper nourishment and revolt against the heart; if the pericardium is weak, the heart will be attacked and the nourishing activities of the triple warmer will be less effective.

One main function of this meridian is to protect the heart – physically as well as energetically. The pericardium is a fibrous sac enclosing a slippery lubricated membrane which prevents friction as the heart beats. Stresses and shocks first affect the pericardium and do not penetrate the heart unless the pericardium is weakened.

Triple Warmer/Endocrine/Three E Meridian
Yang Meridian
Partner Meridian – Pericardium – Yin
Element – Fire
Organ Maximum Energy Period – 9 pm to 11 pm

The triple warmer meridian governs the cycle of ch'i trans-formation. This is the partner of the circulation meridian and thus works closely with it. Though there is no anatomical organ that correlates with the triple warmer, the Chinese believe that all the organs in the body are guarded by it and that heat is controlled by this function.

The three 'heaters' or 'warmers' correspond to divisions of the torso; the upper warmer to the thoracic cavity; the middle warmer to the abdominal cavity; the lower warmer to the pelvic cavity. This meridian governs activities involving all the organs; it unites the respiratory, digestive and excretory functions into an energetic whole. It may be related to the hypothalamus, the link between the nervous system and

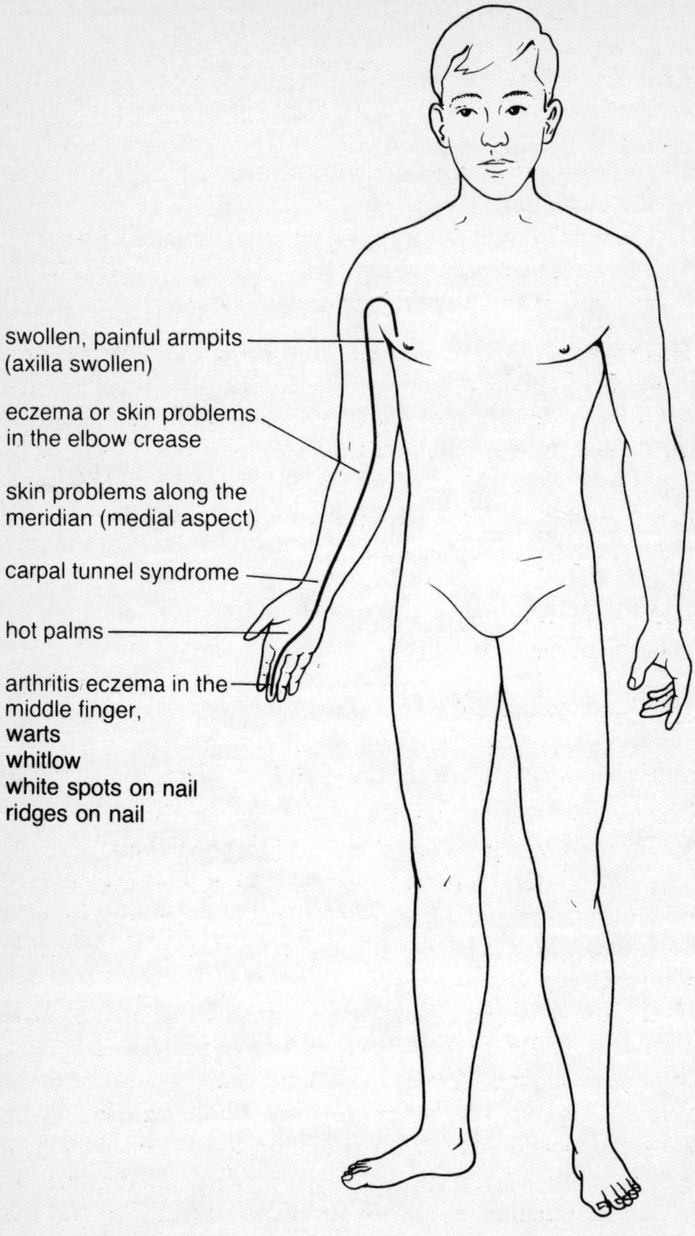

swollen, painful armpits
(axilla swollen)

eczema or skin problems
in the elbow crease

skin problems along the
meridian (medial aspect)

carpal tunnel syndrome

hot palms

arthritis eczema in the
middle finger,
warts
whitlow
white spots on nail
ridges on nail

Fig. 11. The circulation/pericardium meridian

endocrine glands. Its functions include:

1. Regulation of the autonomic nervous system and thus of the heart and abdominal organs especially in their response to emotion.
2. Control of the pituitary gland (which regulates output of all the endocrine glands).
3. Regulation of body temperature, appetite and thirst.
4. Control of emotions and moods – the urges of pleasure and displeasure which influence social relations.

This meridian, like its partner, has several names, as it is tied to numerous organs. In English it is called the triple warmer, in Chinese *sanjiao* which means three body cavity – signifying the division of the body into three sections. The burner of the upper section, the breast cavity, is the lungs; the middle burner in the diaphragm section is the spleen/pancreas; the burners of the lower pelvic section are the kidneys.

Gall Bladder Meridian
Yang Meridian
Partner Meridian – Liver – Yin
Element – Wood
Organ Maximum Energy Period – 11 pm to 1 am

It is essential to note that the Chinese think about the organs as functions operating on all levels of the body-mind . . . 'the liver has the functions of a military leader who excels in his strategic planning; the gall bladder occupies the position of an important and upright official who excels through his decisions and judgment' (Nei Ching).

According to the Ancients the attitudes of all the other organs originate in the energy of the gall bladder. It is different from the other hollow organs in that all the others transport 'impure' or foreign matter – food, liquids and the waste products thereof. Only the gall bladder transports 'pure' liquids exclusively, in that it stores and concentrates bile.

This meridian is one of the most well-travelled meridians, traversing almost the entire body except the arms. It zigzags throughout the head in a pattern which, in times of stress and

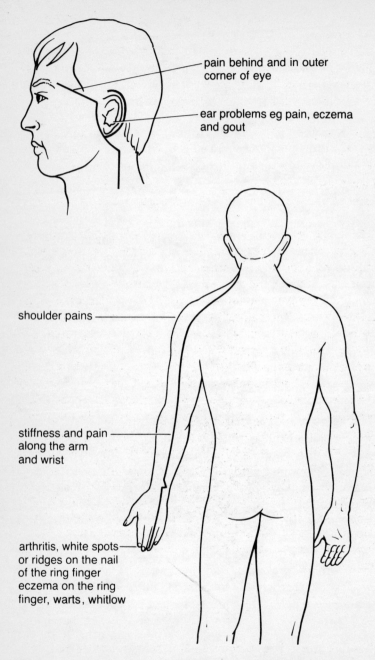

pain behind and in outer corner of eye

ear problems eg pain, eczema and gout

shoulder pains

stiffness and pain along the arm and wrist

arthritis, white spots or ridges on the nail of the ring finger eczema on the ring finger, warts, whitlow

Fig. 12. The triple warmer/endocrine/three E meridian

tension, becomes like a vice and is therefore important in cases of headaches, neck tension and 'uptightness'.

The *Nei Ching* says that the gall bladder rules decision making, thus anger and rash decisions may be due to an excess of gall bladder ch'i, while indecision and timidity may be a sign of gall bladder disharmony and weakness.

Liver Meridian
Yin Meridian
Partner Meridian – Gall Bladder – Yang
Element – Wood
Organ Maximum Energy Period – 1 am to 3 am

'The liver rules flowing and spreading' according to the Chinese classics. The liver or liver ch'i is responsible for the smooth movement of bodily substances and for the regularity of body activities. It moves the ch'i and blood in all directions, sending them to every part of the body. The *Nei Ching* metaphorically calls the liver 'the general of an army' because it maintains evenness and harmony of movement throughout the body.

The liver is the primary centre of metabolism. Not only does it secrete bile, synthesize proteins, neutralize toxins and regulate blood sugar levels, it also stores glycogen (starch), changes it back into glucose (sugar) and releases it when needed. Since the brain does not store any glucose, the liver's steady supply is crucial to life, and this is why the Chinese saw the liver as vital to conscious and unconscious thought processes.

The liver meridian helps control the functions of the nervous system and is very important for psychological problems such as depression and anger. Motivation – the will to become 'that self which one truly is' . . . is associated with balance of this meridian along with a sense of well-being and a reasonable temperament.

CASE HISTORIES

A reflexologist is a therapist who, by stimulating reflexes in the feet, encourages the body to heal itself. In most

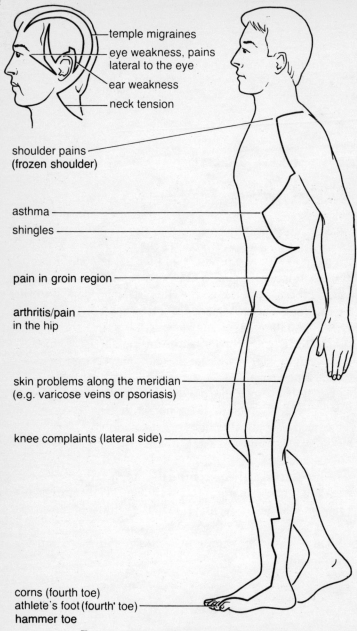

temple migraines

eye weakness, pains lateral to the eye

ear weakness

neck tension

shoulder pains (frozen shoulder)

asthma

shingles

pain in groin region

arthritis/pain in the hip

skin problems along the meridian (e.g. varicose veins or psoriasis)

knee complaints (lateral side)

corns (fourth toe)
athlete's foot (fourth' toe)
hammer toe

Fig. 13. The gall bladder meridian

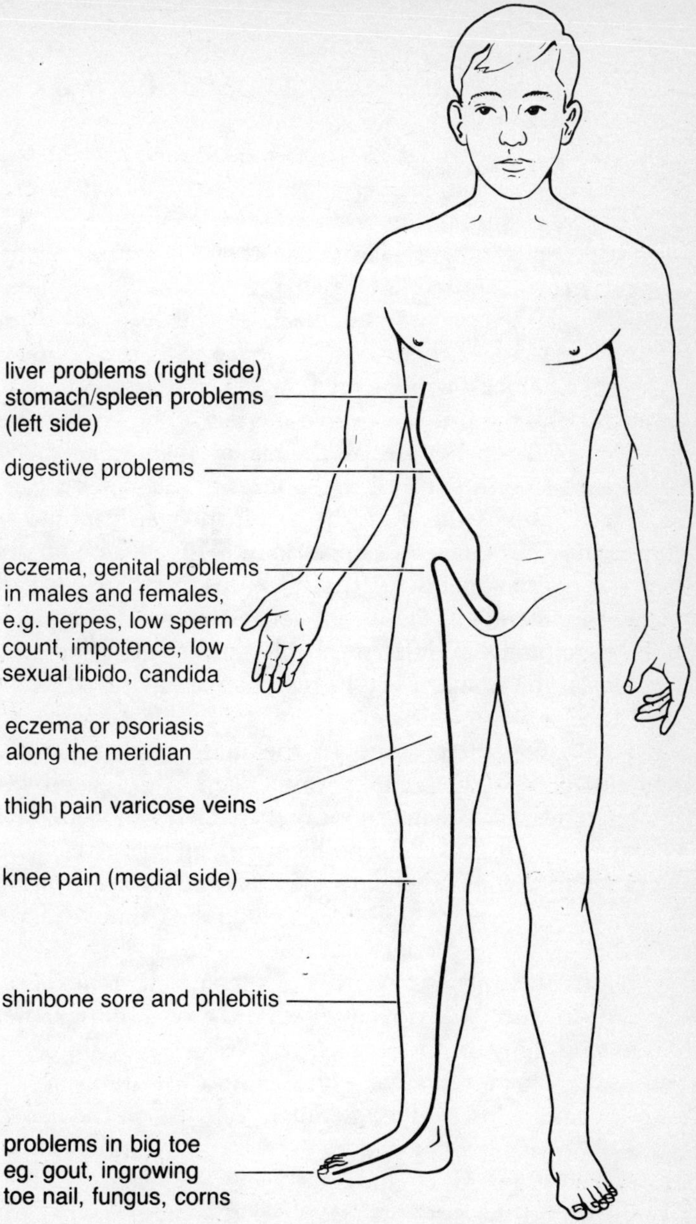

liver problems (right side)
stomach/spleen problems
(left side)

digestive problems

eczema, genital problems
in males and females,
e.g. herpes, low sperm
count, impotence, low
sexual libido, candida

eczema or psoriasis
along the meridian

thigh pain varicose veins

knee pain (medial side)

shinbone sore and phlebitis

problems in big toe
eg. gout, ingrowing
toe nail, fungus, corns

Fig. 14. The liver meridian

countries reflexologists are not allowed to diagnose any specific condition. In my work as a teacher and practitioner I have found it important that a client understands the nature of their complaints so that they are more willing to cooperate with any advice. In order to understand the complaint the practitioner requires a detailed case history of all symptoms, not only those causing the most severe problems at the time of consultation. The complaints can then be related to the meridians in order to ascertain which organs are out of balance. Instead of using the symptoms to diagnose a medical condition one must understand them in accordance with the Chinese philosophy of blockage in energy flow.

Study of the path of the twelve meridians shows that the stomach meridian penetrates all the major organs in the body as well as passing through all the reflexes of the major organs in the feet. This is therefore the dominant meridian and it is often the root cause of congestions. This will obviously affect the partner meridian, the spleen/pancreas, as well as all the other meridians. This root congestion will manifest as different symptoms in different people, but in ninety percent of problems, the stomach and its meridian are involved.

In the case histories where there are problems with the arms and hands these relate to the lung, large intestine, circulation/pericardium, triple warmer/endocrine, small intestine and heart meridians. None of these meridians penetrate any of the major organs, but a problem with an organ can cause a blockage in the ch'i energy in the arms and hands resulting in uncomfortable symptoms – for example the painful thumbs mentioned in the first two case histories.

It is of vital importance to do a complete reflexology treatment in each case, no matter what the symptoms, rather than to work only on the isolated reflexes one may think are congested. Weakness may be expressed in congestions of ch'i energy at any point along a meridian, not just in the actual organs. For example in the case histories relating to the large intestine meridian the main symptoms were manifest in problems on the arms and face, yet the cause was a large intestine imbalance. The kidney and bladder meridians are partner meridians and the main symptoms which indicate imbalance in these organs are headaches, weak eyes, neck tension and back problems and, to some degree, sciatica and leg problems. Dis-ease in the liver and gall bladder meridians often manifest as migraines, gout, nausea, gall stones, frozen shoulder, hip and leg complaints and sexual problems.

The following case histories have all been effectively treated with the reflexology techniques described in this book in Chapter 6. The techniques clear the congestions in the meridians allowing the energy to flow freely and the body to reach a state of balance. Each case history has been described so that the reader can relate the most painful symptoms to blockages along specific meridians but, as previously mentioned, one will inevitably find numerous symptoms relating to the stomach, spleen and pancreas and their meridians. Therefore a change in diet and lifestyle will always have positive results.

Lung Meridian (See illustration p. 33)
Female: Age – 30s
Symptoms: The main reason the client came for treatment was severe pain in a 'nerve' in both thumbs. Other symptoms noted: feels a 'total mess' – allergies; skin problems; rashes on her face and scalp; frequently blocked nose; headaches (forehead and neck); wine makes her nauseous; discontinued contraceptive pills three to four months previously – periods are now regular but heavy and painful; suffers slight constipation.

On studying the case history, one notices obvious symptoms related to the stomach, spleen/pancreas and their meridians – such as allergies, rashes on her face, heavy and painful periods and slight constipation. But the reason she sought treatment was due to the problem with her thumbs which indicates a blockage in the ch'i energy of the lung meridian.

Female: Age – 60s
Symptoms: The main problem, extremely painful thumbs, had been previously diagnosed as arthritis. Other symptoms include bronchial problems; 'nervous' throat – she is constantly clearing her throat; and chronic constipation.

Large callouses on the lung and bronchi reflexes of her feet indicate problems in the respiratory system, while the pain in her thumbs verifies this.

As mentioned in the introduction, problems with the stomach, spleen/pancreas and their meridians are often the root cause and this also applied in this case. Reference to the stomach meridian shows that the pathway includes the bronchi, lung, throat and large intestine. But the main congestion in the ch'i energy is related to the lung meridian.

Large Intestine (Colon) Meridian (See illustration p. 34)
Female: Age – 38
Symptoms: As a teenager she had a wart on her right index finger. She suffered from cold sores on the lips and inside the nose four times a year for which treatment was required. Constipation; nervous stomach which would progress into painful colic if left unattended. Colds invariably developed into chest problems and occasionally pneumonia. As soon as she disrupts her diet she develops fever blisters on her lips and sores in her nose, and the wart scar becomes sore and itchy. These are all symptoms found along the large intestine meridian and when the sores erupt they are warning signals of overloading this organ.

Again none of the meridians in the arm and face penetrate any major organs. But organs related to the meridians in the arms – in this case the large intestine – are penetrated by the stomach and other meridians and the cause will therefore usually be found in one or more of the major organs and their meridians.

Female: Age – mid 50s
Symptoms: Pain in upper right arm from forearm to index finger. The arm sometimes goes into spasm. This condition has existed for three years. Neck tension; constipation (takes laxatives regularly); slow digestion; had a hiatus hernia; meningitis as a child; one short leg; backache.
Previous Operations: Appendectomy and an operation for endiometriosis.

As in the previous case, the main problems were with her arms which indicate congestions along the large intestine meridian. However, one still needs to study and stimulate all other organs and their meridians.

Stomach Meridian (See illustration p. 35)
Female: Age – 55
Symptoms: The reason she sought treatment was a continuous laryingitis problem which had occured six times in one year. Other symptoms noted include fatigue, constipation and tension headaches.
Previous Operations: Appendectomy; hysterectomy; lumpectomy from breast under nipple.

These symptoms all run along the stomach meridian except the tension headaches which relate to the bladder meridian. The hysterectomy can be seen as caused by a combination of meridians – the stomach and the spleen/pancreas.

This is a classic example of a ch'i energy imbalance along the stomach meridian. Over the years symptoms have been dealt with by operations and medication. However, the main cause, an imbalance in the acid/alkaline intake in food, had not been considered.

Female: Age – 30s
Symptoms: The client's main concerns were a constant 'burning' stomach, the bad condition of her nails and dry hair. Other symptoms noted include fatigue, slight constipation, regular menstrual cycle but heavy and painful with sore breasts and backache. Generally has very bad teeth.
Previous Operations: Tonsillectomy; wisdom teeth extracted.

The 'burning stomach' was a sure sign of an acid condition. Her food intake consisted mainly of diet coke, coffee, cheese, bread and pasta and she ate very few vegetables. It is therefore understandable that the stomach and its meridian are the cause, but other symptoms have manifested as well to indicate the congestion. The hair, nails and fatigue can be related to the thyroid (on the stomach meridian). The large intestine (constipation) and teeth are also on the stomach meridian. The breasts were sore on the sides (pancreas meridian) and this links with the heavy cycle.

Spleen/Pancreas Meridian (See illustration p.38)
Female: Age – 40s
Symptoms: Daily headaches; constipation; sweet tooth; regular menstrual cycle but heavy with slight cramps.
Previous Operations: Bunion removed: lumpectomy on right breast.

The client's main problem was daily headaches which indicate an imbalance on the bladder meridian. I considered this case to be more of a problem with the spleen/pancreas and its meridian as the other symptoms and operations noted were largely on the spleen/pancreas meridian. However, the effect of the imbalance was manifest in the form of headaches.

Female: Age – late 20s.
Symptoms: Chronic skin problems on the face; system feels 'burny'; constipation; headaches; painful menstruation until she started taking contraceptive pills three months previously.
Previous Operations: Bunions removed.

This is a combination of problems along the stomach and spleen/pancreas meridians. The bunion problem was an early indication of an imbalance in the pancreas, but as the cause was not treated, the problems moved on to the stomach and resulted in skin and digestive problems. The headaches are due to congestions on the bladder meridian.

Heart Meridian (See illustration p.40)
Female: Age – 62
Symptoms: Medical diagnosis of a weak heart – has an 'extra tick'; pain in little finger on the left hand; aching muscles on the left side of the body specifically the left shoulder which can last up to three to four weeks; middle-ear imbalance. (Refer to illustration of the heart meridian and its partner the small intestine – pages 40 and 41.) Other symptoms noted: constipation; nausea which continues at times for up to three weeks; instant migraines after eating cheese or chocolate; high blood pressure; problems with menstrual cycle – still has periods despite her age and had cramps which stopped when she started taking contraceptive pills.
Previous Operations: Appendectomy; bunion removal twenty

years before; three cysts removed from the breast (on the pancreas meridian).

Although there are numerous problems relating to the heart meridian, I believe the main cause is on the stomach and spleen/pancreas meridians – obvious in the problems with the menstrual cycle, three cysts, bunions and appendectomy. The liver and gall bladder are also penetrated by the stomach meridian which could produce the symptoms of nausea and migraines. Note also that the kidneys are on the stomach meridian and the heart is on the kidney meridian. To take care of a weak heart, one should not overload the kidneys. This can be prevented by ensuring correct acid/alkaline balance in food intake.

Small Intestine Meridian (See illustration p.41)
Female: Age – early 30s
Symptoms: Severe neck, back and shoulder problems – pinched sensation from shoulder down the arm and at one point she lost all feeling in her arm; weak stomach – often experiences cramps after meals; weakness in throat; tennis elbow; at the age of six had a hernia in the groin; at age five suffered a severe ear infection which caused balance problems.

Problems along the small intestine meridian are obvious in the symptoms on the shoulder, neck/arm, elbow, ears and throat. Again remember that meridians in the arms do not penetrate any major organs and one would have to look for the cause on one of the main meridians and the related organs. The weak stomach and cramps after meals indicate a stomach imbalance. But the ch'i energy congestions are mainly located along the arm, shoulder, neck, ears and throat.

Female: Age – late 30s
Symptoms: The client was recommended by her doctor to try reflexology for the very painful trigenimous neuralgia in her face. After ten years of medical treatment, the only further relief they could offer was to sever the nerve in the face which would cause paralysis on one side. Other symptoms noted: Bloated painful colon with constipation and diarrhoea; bleeding gums; heavy menstrual cycle which lasts over eight

days; was on excessive medication – nine painkillers a day plus sleeping tablets.

The first problem to solve would be the constipation. The neuralgia is obviously a symptom of an imbalance of the small intestine and its meridian. A side-effect of the medication is constipation so it is a vicious circle.

Bladder Meridian (See illustration p.43)
Female: Age – 40s
Symptoms: Headaches in the crown, forehead and neck region; backaches; constantly tired; high blood pressure; was a bedwetter.
Previous Operations: Ureter stretched; hysterectomy; operations on both knees with the result that she cannot bend her knees at all.

The headaches and backaches can be traced to the bladder meridian while all the operations are situated on the stomach and spleen/pancreas meridians.

Male: Age – 50s
Symptoms: Daily migraines which run from the back of the head over the crown; generally feels stressed at work and at home; doesn't sleep well – has to relieve himself three to four times a night; fatigue.
Previous Operations: Appendectomy; tonsillectomy; prostate operation.

The appendix and tonsils are on the stomach meridian, whereas the prostate is on the spleen/pancreas meridian. Feeling stressed, bad sleep patterns and fatigue are the result of an imbalance on the stomach and spleen/pancreas meridians. The effects – headaches and weak bladder – are found on the bladder meridian.

Kidney Meridian (See illustration p.44)
Male: Age – mid 60s
Symptoms: General bad circulation; painful calves; tingling burning sensation on the feet; has to get up every night to urinate.
Previous Operations: Three bypass operations; lumpectomy on the elbow.

Reference to the kidney meridian shows that the heart is situated on its pathway. The burning area on the feet was around the kidney reflexes. Furthermore, five plantar warts were situated on the heart reflex of his foot. The lump on the elbow can be traced to the heart meridian. Problems with the calf muscles relate to the partner meridian, the bladder.

Circulation/Pericardium Meridian (See illustration p.46)
I have only seen case histories along the pericardium meridian as symptoms within larger case histories. Lesser symptoms such as eczema, psoriasis, pains in the armpits, carpal tunnel syndrome and arthritis in the middle finger have all been periphery problems of imbalances along the stomach, spleen/pancreas or kidney meridians. Other symptoms which are a result of an imbalance along the pericardium meridian are heart disease; disturbances in heart rhythm; mental disorders such as fear, nervousness and schizophrenia; car sickness and nausea.

Triple Warmer/Endocrine/Three E Meridian (See illustration p.48)
Female: Age – early 30s
Symptoms: Severe eczema on both ring fingers – cannot wear rings; prolapsed uterus – doctor recommended a hysterectomy after a difficult birth.
Previous Operations: Tonsillectomy; appendectomy; lumpectomy on breast around nipple area.

All the symptoms and operations are a result of imbalances along the stomach and spleen/pancreas meridians. The effects of the imbalances have manifest as severe eczema on the ring fingers – the endocrine meridian.

Female: Age – early 40s.
Symptoms: Pains around the ears – diagnosed by her GP as gout – had been so severe she was not able to wash or comb her hair or lie on her ear, particularly during menstruation or ovulation; menstrual cycle problems; sore breasts; weakness in the throat.

This client drank red wine with her meals every evening which affected the endocrine meridian so severely that it resulted in gout. Menstrual cycle problems relate to the spleen/pancreas meridian and the sore breast and weakness in the throat relate to its partner the stomach meridian.

Gall Bladder Meridian (See illustration p.50)
Female: Age – 50s
Symptoms: Depression and nervousness; pain in the right knee extending up to the hip joint – mainly affecting her during the night; acidic burning urine; previous kidney problems; headaches on the temple and top of the head; pain around the ears; heavy menstruation although at menopause age; hot flushes; slight constipation.

The client came for treatment for depression and nervousness. This can sometimes be seen as an imbalance in the pancreas and therefore tied in with the spleen/pancreas and stomach and their meridians. The other symptoms noted – headaches, pain around the ears and pain in the knee relate to the gall bladder meridian. The previous kidney problems, acidic burning urine, heavy menstruation, hot flushes and slight constipation can also be related to the stomach and spleen/pancreas and their meridians.

Female: Age – 50s
Symptoms: Severe lower back pain; leg pains on lateral side; constipation; nausea (cannot tolerate rich foods); allergic to painkillers; hyperventilates; very acidic; sore gums; regular menstrual cycle but painful and heavy.

Previous Operations: Gall stones removed twenty years before.

The leg pains are on the gall bladder meridian but the acidity, constipation, problems with gall stones and sore gums are all on the stomach meridian.

Liver Meridian (See illustration p.51)
Female: Age – 50s
Symptoms: Low libido since hysterectomy two years previously; skin problems; weak bladder; eyes have weakened since a bladder repair operation.

The libido and hysterectomy are related to an imbalance on the liver meridian, but the hysterectomy could be related to the spleen/pancreas. Notice the link between the eyes and the bladder.

Female: Age – 60s
Symptoms: Gout in big toe; occasional nausea; medial knee pains; neck calcified; loose stomach; irregular menstrual cycle when younger which was heavy and painful; had difficulty becoming pregnant; occasional hot flushes.
Previous Operations: Appendectomy; ovarian cysts removed.

The gout and knee pains are on the liver meridian. The irregular menstrual cycle is related to the pancreas while the partner meridian – the stomach – is evident in the operations.

4

Mapping The Feet

UNDERSTANDING THE STRUCTURE of the feet in relation to the body is the first and most important step to understanding reflexology. It is, in fact, very simple, as the feet are a perfect microcosm or mini-map of the whole body and all the organs and body parts are reflected on the feet in almost the same arrangement as in the body. These reflexes are found on the soles, tops and along the inside and outside of the feet and their positions follow a logical anatomical pattern similar to that of the body.

MAPPING THE REFLEXES ON THE FEET

The body itself can be considered as divided horizontally into four parts: the head and neck area; the thoracic area from the shoulders to the diaphragm; the abdominal area from the diaphragm to the pelvic area, and the pelvis. These areas can be clearly delineated on the feet and provide a precise picture of the body as it is reflected on the feet. We will therefore examine the situation of body organs in horizontal divisions, as this facilitates easy study and reference. It also fits in more accurately with the massage technique I teach, which is easier to understand if it is studied together with the meridians.

The sections described above are also clearly visible in the foot structure:

1. The head and neck area = the toes
2. The thoracic area = the ball of the foot
3. The abdominal area = the arch
4. The pelvic area = the heel
5. The reproductive area = the ankle:
6. The spine = the inner foot
7. The outer body = the outer foot
8. Breast area and special circulation points = the tops of the feet.

The Head and Neck Area – The Toes

The toes incorporate reflexes to all parts of the body found above the shoulder girdle. If you imagine the two big toes as two half heads with a common neck the positions of the reflexes are placed very logically. Obviously some reflexes overlap as they do in the body. Each big toe contains reflex points for the pituitary gland, pineal gland, hypothalamus, brain, temples, teeth, the seven cervical (neck) vertebrae, sinuses, mastoid, tonsils, nose, mouth and other face reflexes as well as part of the eustachian tubes.

The other four toes on each foot contain reflex points for the eyes, ears, teeth, sinuses, lachrymal glands (tear ducts), speech centre, upper lymph system, collar bone (shoulder girdle), eustachian tubes, 'chronic' eye and ear problems.

The Head and the Brain
Reflexes of the head and the brain are on the pads of the big toes from the tip behind the nail down over the metatarsal bone; reflexes for the sides of the head and brain are on the sides of the big toes. On the top of the toes are the face reflexes including the mouth, nose, teeth and tonsils. At the base of the big toe are the neck reflexes.

The Sinuses
The sinuses are cavities within the skull bones situated above and to the sides of the nose in the cheekbones behind the

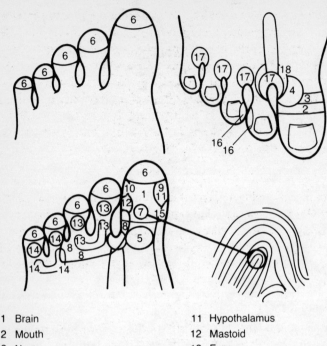

1 Brain
2 Mouth
3 Nose
4 Tonsils
5 Neck
6 Sinus, Teeth and Top of Head
7 Pituitary gland
8 Eustachian gland
9 Pineal gland
10 Temples

11 Hypothalamus
12 Mastoid
13 Eyes
14 Ears
15 Cervical spine (C1–C7)
16 Lachrymal glands
   (tearducts)
17 Upper lymph system
18 Speech centre

Fig. 15. The head and neck area

eyebrows. They communicate with the nasal cavities through small openings. They act as protection for the eyes and the brain and give resonance to the voice.

The reflexes are situated on the tips of all the toes.

The Pituitary Gland
This gland, known also as the 'master gland', is considered the most important gland in the body as it controls the functions of all the endocrine glands. About the size and shape of a cherry, the pituitary gland is attached to the base of the brain. Numerous

hormones are produced by this gland – these influence growth, sexual development, metabolism, pregnancy, mineral and sugar contents of the blood, fluid retention and energy levels.

The reflex point is found on both feet where the whorl of the toe print converges into a central point. It is usually situated on the inner side of the toe and often requires a little searching. More often than not, this reflex is found to be off-centre. Since the hormonal system is extremely sensitive and easily thrown off-balance, this reflex is usually very tender.

The Hypothalamus

A number of bodily activities are controlled by this part of the brain. It regulates the autonomic nervous system and controls emotional reactions, appetite, body temperature and sleep.

The hypothalamus reflex areas are found on both feet on the outer side and top of the big toe – the same reflex point as the pineal gland.

The Pineal Gland

The pineal gland is a small gland situated within the hypothalamus section of the brain. Its functions are not completely understood, but it is known to stimulate the cells in the skin to produce the black pigment melanin. It is thought to play a part in mood and circadian rhythms, and is sometimes referred to as the psychic 'third eye'.

The reflexes are on both feet on the outer tip of the big toes – the same as the hypothalamus reflex.

The Teeth

The reflexes to the teeth are exactly distributed over the ten toes: incisors (1) on the big toe: incisors and canine teeth (2, 3) on the second toe: premolars (4, 5) on the third toe: molars (6, 7) on the fourth toe: wisdom teeth (8) on the fifth toe. These reflexes are in the same position as the sinus reflexes.

The Eyes

The eyes are important sensory organs – the organs of sight. The retina receives impressions of images via the pupils and the lens. The optic nerve conveys the impressions from the receptors in the eye to the visual area of the cerebral cortex where they are interpreted.

These reflexes are on both feet on the cushions of the second and third toes and may extend slightly down the toes. Reflexes for chronic eye conditions are on the 'shelf' at the base of these two toes.

The Ears
The ear is the organ of hearing. It is a highly complex system of cavities, bones and membranes, constructed in such a way that sound waves in the atmosphere are caught up and transmitted to the hearing centre in the temporal lobe of the cerebral cortex. The ear also plays a part in maintaining balance.

The reflexes are situated on both feet on the cushions of the fourth and fifth toes and may extend slightly down the toes. The reflexes for the eustachian tubes extend from the inner side of the big toe along the base of the second and third toes to the fourth toe. Reflexes for chronic ear conditions are found on the 'shelf' at the base of these two toes – the same section as the eustachian tubes. The mastoid – the part of the skull behind the ear which contains the air spaces that communicate with the ear – is also treated on these reflexes.

The Tonsils
These are paired organs composed of lymphatic tissue and thought to be involved in defence of this area. The reflexes are found on both feet – on the top of the foot at the base of the big toe near the web between the big and second toes.

The Lymph System
The lymphatic system forms a subsidiary or secondary circulatory system. It is a network of lymphatic vessels situated throughout the body which acts to drain tissue fluid surrounding the cells in the body. Lymph nodes filter the lymph to prevent infection passing into the blood stream and add lymphocytes which are important for the formation of antibodies and immunological reactions. The main sites of the lymph nodes are in the neck, armpit, thorax, abdomen, groin, pelvis and behind the knee.

On the front of the foot, the webs between the toes are the

reflexes for the drainage of the lymphatics in the neck/chest region of the body. Lymph reflexes for the groin area are tied in with the reproductive system and are found in the same area as the reflexes for the fallopian tubes and vas deferens described later in this chapter. These reflexes run across the top of the foot from the inner ankle bone to the outer ankle bone and incorporate the six main meridians. Congestions in the groin can be traced to a specific meridian and its organ depending on where lumps are situated – proving the significance of the meridians.

The Thoracic Area – The Ball of the Foot

This section of the foot corresponds with the thoracic area in the body from the shoulder girdle to the diaphragm. Several vital reflexes are situated here: the heart, lungs, oesophagus, trachea, bronchi, thyroid and thymus glands, diaphragm and solar plexus.

The Lungs

The lungs are cone-shaped, spongy organs in the thorax which lie on either side of the heart. It is here that the process of respiration takes place – the exchange of oxygen for carbon dioxide. The main air passage of the respiratory system found in the thorax is the trachea (windpipe) which divides into the bronchi to enter the left and right lungs.

The lung reflexes are found on the soles of both feet from the second toe (stomach meridian) to just past the fourth toe (gall bladder meridian). Reflexes of the trachea and bronchi are found below the big toe and second toes (stomach and liver meridians) connected to the lung reflex. These same reflexes are also found in similar positions on the tops of the feet.

The Heart

The heart is a hollow, cone-shaped, muscular organ which lies in the chest on the left side of the body in a space between the lungs. It acts as a pump circulating blood throughout the body. Efficient functioning of the heart is essential to allow good blood circulation throughout the body, which is necessary for efficient transport of gases, foods and waste products. The chest area also contains other major vessels leading to and from the heart – the vena cavae, aorta and other arteries and veins.

The reflex to the heart is situated on the sole of the left foot only – on the kidney meridian above the diaphragm level.

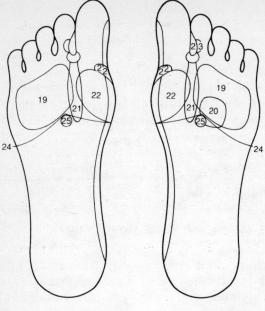

19 Lungs
20 Heart
21 Oesophagus, Trachea, Bronchi, Thymus gland
22 Thyroid, Parathyroid

23 Thyroid–helper reflex (stomach meridian)
24 Diaphragm
25 Solar Plexus

Fig. 16. The thoracic area

The Thymus Gland, Oesophagus, Trachea and Bronchi

The thymus gland is situated in the thoracic cavity. It is quite large in childhood, reaches maximum size at ten to twelve years, then slowly regresses and has almost disappeared in adult life. It is involved in the immune system. Its only known function is the formation of lymphocytes.

The oesophagus is the gullet – a muscular tube passing from the pharynx down through the chest, and joining the stomach below the diaphragm. Food and fluid are propelled through it by peristalsis.

The trachea is the windpipe. It passes down from the larynx into the throat, where it divides into two main bronchi.

The bronchi are the two main divisions of the trachea which enter the lungs.

All these reflexes are found on both feet in the same area – on the soles of the feet in a vertical line between the first and second toes.

The Thyroid Gland
The thyroid gland is located in the neck. It controls the rate of metabolism, which is necessary for normal mental and physical development and maintains the correct amount of calcium in the blood.

This reflex is situated on both feet at the base of the big toe, down around the ball and into the groove below the bone. The most important part is the section along the bone. There is also a 'helper' reflex on the second toe – the stomach meridian.

The Parathyroid Glands
These are four small glands situated around the thyroid gland. Their main function is to maintain the correct amount of calcium and phosphorus in the blood and bones.

The reflex is situated on both feet at the base of the big toe on the outer side.

The Diaphragm
The diaphragm, one of the muscles of respiration, is a large, dome-shaped wall which separates the thorax from the abdomen. It is the most important muscle for breathing.

This reflex is situated on the soles of both feet, and extends across all six meridians at the base of the ball of the foot separating the ball from the arch.

The Solar Plexus
The solar plexus is a network of sympathetic nerve ganglia in the abdomen and is the nerve supply to the abdominal organs below the diaphragm. It is sometimes referred to as the 'abdominal brain' or the 'nerve switchboard' and is situated behind the stomach and in front of the diaphragm.

The reflex is at the same level as the reflex to the diaphragm located at a specific point in the centre of the diaphragm reflex. This point is visible on the foot as the apex of the arch that runs across the base of the ball of the foot. This reflex is most useful for inducing a relaxed state. It can relieve stress and nervousness, aid deep regular breathing and restore calm.

The Abdominal Area – The Arch of the Foot

The arch of the foot is clearly visible on the sole – the raised area which extends from the base of the ball to the beginning of the heel. It is divided into two parts: the upper part corresponds to the section of the body from the diaphragm to the waistline; the lower part corresponds to the section of the body from the waistline to the pelvic area.

Reflexes above the waistline: liver, gall bladder, stomach, pancreas, duodenum, spleen, adrenals and kidneys.

The Liver

The liver is the largest and most complex organ/gland in the body. It controls many of the chemical processes and has many functions. These include: processing nutrients from the blood, storing fats, sugars and proteins until the body needs them; detoxifying the blood and manufacturing bile for fat digestion; storing sugars in the form of glycogen to be used when the body needs an increased supply of energy; and the storage and metabolism of fats and proteins.

This reflex is found on the sole of the right foot only, below the diaphragm level, extending from the pancreas meridian on the inside of the foot to below the little toe. It ends just above the waistline.

The Gall Bladder

This is a small, muscular, pear-shaped sac attached to the under-surface of the liver. Its function is to excrete bile for food digestion.

The gall bladder reflex is on the sole of the right foot only, embedded within the liver reflex beneath and between the third and fourth toes.

The Stomach

The stomach is a large muscular bag which lies below the diaphragm mainly to the left side of the body. Food passes from the mouth down the oesophagus into the stomach where it is churned up and mixed with gastric juices and enzymes to start the digestive process.

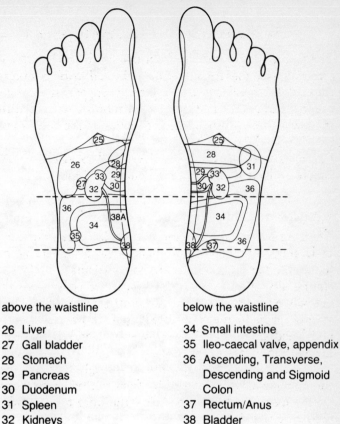

above the waistline	below the waistline
26 Liver	34 Small intestine
27 Gall bladder	35 Ileo-caecal valve, appendix
28 Stomach	36 Ascending, Transverse,
29 Pancreas	Descending and Sigmoid
30 Duodenum	Colon
31 Spleen	37 Rectum/Anus
32 Kidneys	38 Bladder
33 Adrenals	38A Ureter

Fig. 17. The abdominal area

The reflexes are found on the soles of both feet – extending from the big toe to the second toe on the right foot and the big toe to the outer edge of the fourth toe on the left foot. Horizontally they are situated just below the diaphragm level.

The Pancreas
The pancreas is a large glandular structure in the abdomen. It is both an endocrine and exocrine gland secreting insulin and digestive juices. It is probably best known for its function as an endocrine gland and for the production of the hormones insulin and glucagon which are important in the control of sugar metabolism.

71

The reflexes are situated on the soles of both feet – more on the left foot than the right foot – below the stomach and above the waistline. On the right foot it extends into just below the big toe, and on the left foot as far as the fourth toe.

The Duodenum

This is the first, C-shaped part of the small intestine, about 20 to 25 centimetres long. It extends from the pyloric sphincter of the stomach to the jejunum. Pancreatic and common bile ducts open into it, releasing secretions responsible for the breakdown of food.

The reflexes are on the soles of both feet immediately below the pancreas, touching the waistline and extending inwards to the second toe.

The Spleen

The spleen is a large, very vascular, gland-like but ductless organ found on the left side of the body behind the stomach. It plays an important part in the immune system, and is part of the lymphatic system. It contains lymphatic tissue which manufactures the white blood cells, breaks down old red blood corpuscles and filters the lymph of toxins.

The reflex is found on the outer side of the left foot (opposite the liver reflex on the right foot), beneath the fourth toe (gall bladder meridian), just below the diaphragm line in line with the stomach reflex.

The Kidneys

The kidneys are part of the main excretory system of the body – the urinary system – which collectively refers to the kidneys, ureter tubes, urethra and bladder. They are two bean-shaped organs which filter toxins from the blood, produce urine and regulate the retention of important minerals and water.

The reflexes are found on the soles of both feet positioned just above the waistline on the kidney and stomach meridians, just below the stomach reflex. The right kidney is positioned slightly lower than the left kidney.

The Adrenal Glands

These are two triangular endocrine glands situated on the

upper tip of each kidney. As part of the endocrine system they perform numerous vital functions. The adrenal glands are divided into two distinct regions, the cortex and medulla. The adrenal cortex produces steroid hormones which regulate carbohydrate metabolism and have anti-allergic and anti-inflammatory properties. The cortex also produces hormones which control the reabsorption of sodium and water in the kidneys, as well as the secretion of potassium and the sex hormones testosterone and oestrogen.

The adrenal medulla produces adrenaline and noradrenaline which work in conjunction with the sympathetic nervous system. The output of adrenaline is increased at times of anxiety and stress and is responsible for organ changes in the 'fight-or-flight' situation.

The reflexes are situated on the soles of both feet on top of the kidney reflexes.

The Abdominal Area – The Arch of the Foot

Now we come to the lower part of the arch of the foot, which corresponds to the section of the body from the waistline to the pelvic area (diagram, page 71).
Reflexes below the waistline: small intestine, ileo-caecal valve, appendix, large intestine, adrenals, kidneys, ureters, bladder.

The Small Intestine
This is a muscular tube about 6 to 7 metres in length. It is the main area of the digestive tract where absorption takes place. It leads from the pyloric sphincter of the stomach to the caecum of the large intestine and lies in a coiled position in the abdominal cavity surrounded by the large intestine. The small intestine is divided into three sections – the duodenum, jejunum and the ileum.

The reflex is situated on the soles of both feet, under the large intestine reflex just below the waistline to the end of the arch extending across to below the fourth toe.

The Ileo-Caecal Valve
This valve is situated where the small intestine and large intestine join; it therefore controls the passage of contents of

the small intestine through to the large intestine. It prevents backflow of faecal matter from the large intestine and controls mucous secretions.

The reflex is found on the sole of the right foot below and between the third and fourth toes just above the level of the pelvic floor.

The Appendix

The appendix is a worm-like tube about 9 to 10 centimetres in length with a blind end projecting downwards from the caecum of the large intestine in the lower right part of the abdominal cavity. Located directly below the ileo-caecal valve, it helps lubricate the large intestine, is rich in lymphoid tissue and secretes antibodies.

The reflex is situated only on the sole of the right foot, in the same area as the ileo-caecal valve.

The Large Intestine

This is a tube about 1.5 metres in length. It starts on the right side of the body at the caecum (ileo-caecal valve) and goes up the right side to below the liver where it bends to the left (hepatic flexure) and passes across the abdomen as the transverse colon. At the left side of the abdomen, it bends down below the spleen (splenic flexure) to become the descending colon which passes down the left side of the abdomen. It then turns towards the midline and takes the shape of a double S-shaped bend known as the sigmoid flexure. This leads into the rectum which in turn leads to the anus.

When the residue of food reaches the large intestine it is in fluid form. The function of the large intestine is to remove some of the water and salts by absorption and to convert the waste matter into faeces ready for excretion.

The reflexes are found on the soles of both feet. On the right foot this begins just below the reflex for the ileo-caecal valve and extends upwards (ascending colon), then turns just below the liver reflex to become the transverse colon which extends across the entire foot. It continues across to the left foot and turns just below the spleen reflex to become the descending colon. Just above the pelvic floor it turns again into the sigmoid colon which ends at the reflex of the rectum/anus.

The Ureters

Ureter tubes are muscular tubes about 30 centimetres in length which connect the kidneys and bladder and function as a passageway for urine. There are two tubes, one from each kidney, which pass downwards through the abdomen into the pelvis where they enter the bladder.

The reflexes are situated on the soles of both feet linking the kidney reflexes to the bladder reflexes which are situated on the inner side of the instep. The ureter reflex can often be seen as distinct lines running across the arch.

The Bladder

The bladder is an elastic muscular sac situated in the centre of the pelvis. Urine for excretion passes from the kidneys down the ureters and is stored in the bladder until it is eliminated via the urethra.

The reflexes are found on both feet on the side of the foot below the inner ankle bone on the heel line. This reflex is often clearly visible as a puffy area.

The Pelvic Area – The Heel of the Foot

Few organs are represented here, but this area is of vital importance as all six main meridians traverse the pelvic section of the heel. As a result, many congestions here can be traced to meridians and their organs.

The Sciatic Nerve

This is the largest nerve in the body. It arises from the sacral plexus of nerves formed by the lower lumbar and upper sacral spinal nerves. It runs from the buttocks down the back of the thigh to divide just above the knee into two main branches which supply the lower leg. The sciatic nerve and reflex are found on the soles of both feet – in a band about a third of the way down the pad of the heel extending right across the foot.

The Reproductive Area – The Ankle

The outer ankle contains the ovaries/testes reflexes, and the inner ankle contains the uterus, prostate, vagina and penis

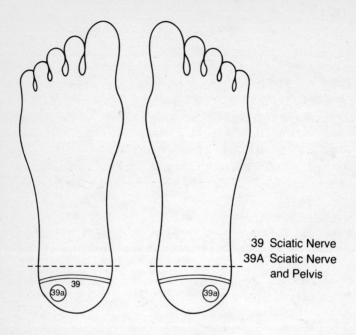

39 Sciatic Nerve
39A Sciatic Nerve
and Pelvis

Fig. 18. The pelvic area

reflexes. The reflex points for the fallopian tubes, lymph drainage area in the groin, vas deferens and seminal vesicles are found in a narrow band running below the outer ankle bone across the top of the foot to the inner ankle bone. The kidney/bladder meridian is situated on both sides up the back of the ankle.

The Ovaries
These are the female gonads or sex glands. They are small, almond-shaped glands about 2 to 3 centimetres long. There are two ovaries – one on each side of the uterus. These are part of the female reproductive system and produce ova as well as the hormones oestrogen and progesterone.

The reflexes are found on both feet on the outer side, midway between the ankle bone and the back of the heel – the right ovary on the right foot, the left ovary on the left foot. The helper area is the heel due to the presence of the meridians.

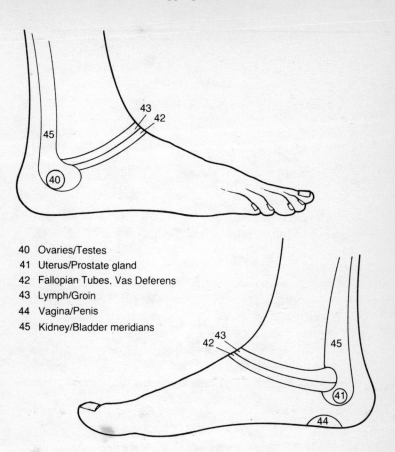

40 Ovaries/Testes
41 Uterus/Prostate gland
42 Fallopian Tubes, Vas Deferens
43 Lymph/Groin
44 Vagina/Penis
45 Kidney/Bladder meridians

Fig. 19. The reproductive area

The Testes

The testes are the male reproductive glands which produce spermatozoa and the male hormone testosterone. There are two testes suspended outside the body in the scrotum – a sac of thin, dark-coloured skin which lies behind the penis.

The reflexes are found on males in the same area as the ovaries in females, that is, midway between the outer ankle bone and the heel. The helper area is the heel.

The Uterus

The uterus is a hollow, pear-shaped organ about 10 centimetres long situated in the centre of the pelvic cavity in females. Its function is the nourishment and protection of the foetus during pregnancy and its expulsion at term.

The reflex points are located on both feet on the inside of the ankles, midway on a diagonal line between the ankle bone and the back of the heel. The helper area is the heel.

The Prostate Gland

This gland lies at the base of the bladder and surrounds the urethra. It produces the thin lubricating fluid which forms part of the semen to aid the transport of sperm cells.

Reflexes are found on both feet in the same place as the uterus reflex on females – midway in a diagonal line between the inner ankle bone and the heel. Again, the heel is the helper area.

The Fallopian Tubes

In females these two tubes, about 10 to 14 centimetres in length, connect the ovaries with the cavity of the uterus. Their function is to conduct the ova expelled from the ovaries during ovulation down the tube to the uterus.

The reflexes are found on both feet. They run across the top of the foot linking the reflex of the uterus to the reflex of the ovaries. This area is usually massaged in conjunction with the reflexes of the ovaries and uterus.

The Seminal Vesicles/Vas Deferens

The seminal vesicles lie next to the prostate and store semen. The vas deferens are a pair of excretory ducts which convey semen from the testes through the prostate and into the urethra.

The reflexes are located in the same area as the fallopian tubes in females – across the top of the foot from one ankle bone to the other, linking the prostate and testes reflexes.

The Spine – The Inner Foot

The inside of each foot is naturally curved to correspond to the spine.

The Spine

The spine, also known as the backbone or vertebral column, is the central support of the body. It carries the weight of the body and is an important axis of movement. The spine is made up of thirty-three vertebrae. The structure of the bones is arranged in such a way as to give the spine four curves. The spine is divided into four sections from top to bottom: seven cervical vertebrae (including the first two, axis and atlas) = the neck; twelve thoracic vertebrae = the back; five lumbar vertebrae = the loin; five sacral vertebrae = the pelvis; four/five coccycal vertebrae = the tail. The vertebrae of the sacrum and coccyx are fused to form two immobile bones. Vertebrae are joined by

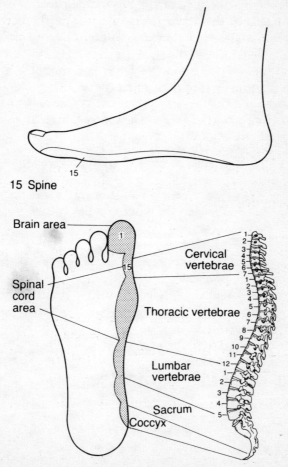

Fig.20. The vertebrae

discs of cartilage and are held in place by ligaments.

The spinal column encloses the spinal cord, the central channel of the nervous system, which is a continuation of the brain stem. It carries the nerves from the brain to all parts of the body. Associated with each vertebra is a spinal nerve. These nerves arise from the spinal cord and affect the level of the body at which they arise – that is, the thoracic nerves affect the thorax, and the lumbar nerves the lower abdomen and legs.

The reflex zones run along the inner side of both feet – half the spine represented on each foot. The cervical vertebrae reflex runs from the base of the big toe nail to the base of the toe (between the first and second joints of the big toe). The thoracic reflex runs along the ball of the foot below the big toe (shoulder to waistline), the arch from the waistline to pelvic line corresponds to the lumbar region and the heel line to the base of the heel to the sacrum/coccyx.

The Outer Foot – The Outer Body

The outer edge of the foot corresponds to the outer part of the body – the joints, ligaments and surrounding muscles. From the base of the toe to the diaphragm line = shoulder and upper arm; diaphragm line to waistline = elbow, forearm, wrist and hand; waistline to end of heel = leg, knee and hip.

The Knee
The knee joint joins the upper and lower leg and facilitates flexibility of the lower limb.

Reflexes are found on both feet on the outer side just below the bony projection of the fifth metatarsal which is usually quite prominent on the side of the foot. Again, remember the six meridians run through the knee, so by pinpointing the exact location of the knee pain, one can relate it to a specific meridian and locate the problematic organ.

The Hip
The hip joint is where the thigh bone (femur) meets the pelvis.

The reflex is found on both feet extending towards the toe in front of the knee reflex. It covers a half moon shape, moving

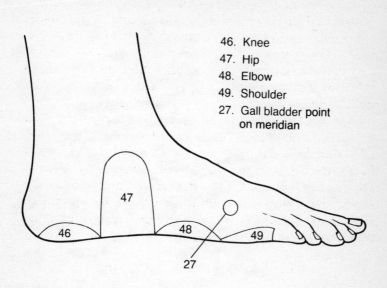

46. Knee
47. Hip
48. Elbow
49. Shoulder
27. Gall bladder point
    on meridian

Fig. 21. The outer foot

out from the line along the side of the foot and up in line with one fourth toe and the gall bladder meridian. A number of hip problems may be gall bladder related, as the gall bladder meridian passes directly through the hip.

The Elbow and Shoulder

The elbow is the joint between the upper arm and the forearm. It is formed by the humerus above and the radius and ulna below. The shoulder joint is where the bone of the upper arm (humerus) meets the shoulder blade (scapula).

The reflexes to the elbow are situated on both feet on the outer side along the arch and the ball. The shoulder and the surrounding muscles are found on both feet at the base of the fifth toe covering the sole, outer side and top.

The Top of the Foot – The Breast Area and Circulation Points

Reflexes found on the top of the foot include the circulation and breast. Most of the reflexes represented on the soles are also found on the tops of the feet in the meridians.

The Breast

Here it is important to look at the meridians. If there are breast problems, note exactly where these are situated so as to identify the meridian that runs through the affected section of the breast and thereby the problem organ.

Special Circulation Points

These points are to stimulate the heart, circulation and body temperature. These are found on the top and soles of both feet at the web between the second and third toes. As these are points on the stomach meridian, they have an effect on the thyroid which in turn affects body temperature, heart and circulation.

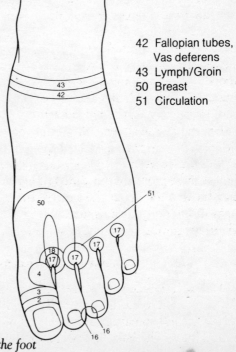

42 Fallopian tubes,
    Vas deferens
43 Lymph/Groin
50 Breast
51 Circulation

Fig. 22. The top of the foot

5

Reading The Feet

THERE IS an overriding tendency to blame foot problems and deformities such as corns, callouses and bunions on ill-fitting shoes. This is part of the problem – but only part. Problem areas on the feet relate to problem areas in the body. Which is the cause and which the effect is questionable. It is a 'chicken or egg' situation. Congestions along a meridian will disrupt the body's equilibrium – be they internal or external. If the problem is internal, the reflex area and the relevant meridian will be particularly sensitive to excess pressure and friction and more susceptible to the formations of corns and callouses. However, these external problems cause congestions along the meridians in the same way as internal congestions. If these are not dealt with they have an adverse effect on body parts along the whole meridian creating an imbalance throughout the body.

With the combination of reflexes and meridians, we can now look at these problems in a different light and unravel the tales they have to tell about the state of the body as a whole. The areas where the problems manifest are particularly significant when integrating the concept of meridians.

Bunions (Hallux valgus)

A bunion (Hallux valgus) is a prominence of the head of the metatarsal bone at its junction with the big toe. It is caused by inflammation and swelling of the bursa (bursitis) at that joint. The bursa is a pocket of fluid enclosed in fibrous

83

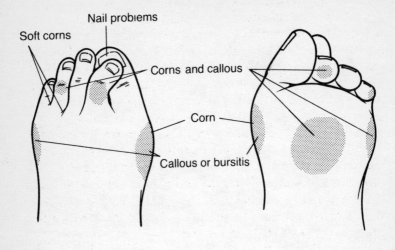

Soft corns

Nail problems

Corns and callous

Corn

Callous or bursitis

Fig. 23. Hammer second toe and other common foot problems

tissue which surrounds the joints and serves to protect them from friction. In this condition the metatarsal joint becomes enlarged and is therefore subject to pressure and friction from shoes which further aggravates the problem and damages the skin.

As the bunion develops, the big toe moves sideways constricting and displacing the other toes – particularly the second toe which is forced out of alignment into a position on top of the big toe. This is known as a hammer toe and it may, in time, become permanently bent. Its position above the other toes makes it prone to corns and callouses on the top of the toe due mainly to pressure from shoes.

The constriction of the toes can also affect the little toe – forcing it towards the middle of the foot and causing a 'bunionette' on the outer side at the base of the little toe.

What Meridians Reveal About Bunions

Two important meridians are found on the big toe – the spleen/pancreas meridian on the outer side and the liver meridian on the inner side towards the second toe. Bunions are situated on the pancreas meridian and the thyroid reflex. The internal branch of the spleen/pancreas meridian runs through the thyroid, further indicating their close relationship. Most people with bunions also have problems along the spleen/pancreas meridian or pancreatic disorders, for example, problems related to sugar metabolism like a sweet tooth; cravings for stimulants like tea, coffee, cigarettes and alchohol, and constant hunger. They may suffer from depression due to the fact that the thyroid is affected. Many people who have had bunions removed or repaired at an early age often develop thyroid problems in later life. Or vice versa – people with thyroid problems often develop bunions. This is because the underlying causes of the symptom – the pancreas and thyroid imbalances – have not been corrected.

Once a bunion has developed in an adult foot it cannot be realigned or straightened without surgery. No exercise or manipulation will push it back. By understanding the connection with the meridians, we can understand the cause of the problem – a pancreas imbalance – and set about rectifying that. This problem is most effectively rectified by a change of diet. Pain caused by bunions can be significantly alleviated with reflexology treatments and a change of diet.

Corns and Callouses

Callouses

Repeated pressure and friction on the skin will cause it to thicken as a means of protection. Foot callouses are quite common as the skin on the feet is subject to a great deal of pressure – particularly from ill-fitting shoes. If this thickening is aggravated by consistent pressure, the build-up of skin will lead to pain and discomfort. Callouses are especially visible on the tops of the toes and soles of the feet. They are easily removed by a chiropodist but will recur if the reason for their formation is not dealt with.

Corns

Corns usually develop on the joints of the toes which, due to their relative prominence, are particularly sensitive to pressure from shoes. At the focal point of this pressure, the skin hardens and thickens. A corn – basically a concentrated area of hard skin – forms in the middle of the area of thickening where the pressure is greatest. Corns also develop on the soles of the feet in areas of excessive pressure. The stabbing pain which is often characteristic of corns is caused by the hard skin exerting secondary pressure onto the sensitive tissue and nerve endings beneath it.

Meridians and Corns and Callouses

Corns and callouses usually develop on the tops of the toes. It is important to note exactly where these appear and establish on which meridian they are manifest and in turn which organs are out of balance. For example, the stomach meridian runs along the second and third toes, and problems here indicate congestions along the stomach meridian. Symptoms such as acidity, gastritis, ulcers, appendix and tonsil trouble, sinus, skin problems and breast problems are often found in people with problems on the second and third toes.

The second and third toes are also often longer than the first toe. This can indicate a genetic weakness in the stomach, often inherited, but can also be due to dietary deficiencies during the embryonic period which have caused stomach weakness. If the weakness is genetic, care should always be taken with diet – for example, avoiding excessively acid foods.

Some people have a long callous under the second toe. This relates to the bronchi/throat reflex area. If there is a deep groove in the skin it could also relate to a weakness in the throat, and the person may have a tendency to suffer from throat, tonsil and bronchial problems. The stomach meridian traverses through the throat area – tonsils, thyroid and the throat itself. The stomach meridian is on top of the second toe while the throat and bronchial reflexes are on the soles between the first and second toes. Moving down, the meridian runs underneath the bone region – the thyroid. Many people have a groove or hard callous around the bone which, again, can be related to an imbalance in the thyroid region; often due to an imbalance in the spleen/pancreas and stomach meridians, as these two are very closely related. Hard skin over the lung reflex is also a common problem. This can indicate a weak chest. The stomach meridian also runs through the lung area and the gall bladder meridian enters the lung area from the side.

As you can see, it is important to take careful note of where corns and callouses form and refer them to the meridians in order to understand the root cause of the problem.

Athlete's Foot

Athlete's foot is a fungal infection which usually manifests on the skin between the toes. This is the most common site of infection as the moist, warm conditions stimulate the fungus to multiply. The fungus thrives on keratin – a protein found in the outer layers of the skin. A major symptom of this condition is itching. If this is accompanied by loose scaley skin surrounding patches of pink, exposed skin, it is a definite sign of infection.

Occasionally a fissure – a split in the skin – may occur at the base of the toes. If this is deep, there could be a problem with bleeding. It could also be infected with bacteria and become inflamed if not taken care of. According to medical belief athlete's foot is very easily transmitted to others, particularly where there is communal bathing.

Meridians and Athlete's Foot

Again, it is important to take note of exactly where on the foot the problem is. Athlete's foot will most often manifest in between the fourth and fifth toes – the bladder meridian – and can therefore be related to the bladder. If between the third and fourth toe, it would be related to the gall bladder meridian.

Toenail Troubles

Ingrowing Toenail

As anyone who suffers from this problem knows, it can be extremely painful and uncomfortable. Interestingly, those most often affected by this condition are young people in their teens and twenties. It usually occurs on the big toe when the side of the nail penetrates the skin of the nail groove and becomes embedded in the soft skin tissue. If the wound is hampered in its efforts to heal, it produces granulation tissue which accumulates on the side and top of the nail. This tissue bleeds very easily. Ingrowing toenails can be caused by cutting the nail too short or cutting down the sides of the nail. Thin brittle nails and moist skin will increase susceptibility to this problem.

Involuted Toenail

An involuted toenail, if not correctly tended, can develop into an ingrowing toenail. This condition occurs when the normal curve of the toenail is so exaggerated that it produces pain down the side of the nail. The exaggerated curve can also encourage the development of corns and callouses on the sides of the nail which will increase discomfort. It is difficult to cut this type of nail, but cutting down the sides must be avoided, as this will result in the new nail growth forcing its way through the soft skin at the side of the nail, causing an ingrowing toenail.

Thickened Toenail

A toenail will thicken if the nail cell production centre is damaged. This can happen if the nail is persistently rubbed against a shoe over a prolonged period, or if the toenail has sustained injury in an accident. Unfortunately, this condition is irreversible. A further complication arises as the nail grows – the new growth curves – and is uncomfortable and unsightly. This curvature is known as a ram's-horn nail. Many elderly people are afflicted by this problem.

Fungal Infection of the Toenail

Fungal infection of the toenail often accompanies athlete's foot. The fungus penetrates the nail causing it to thicken. If the condition deteriorates, the colour and texture of the nail will also be affected, becoming darker and 'crumbly'.

Meridians and Toenail Troubles

With all toenail troubles, it is imperative that meridians are taken into account. Take, for example, ingrowing toenails. This problem is often found in young people and situated on the big toe – the spleen/pancreas meridian mentioned earlier. These people usually have a diet high in sugar, junk food, alcohol, cigarettes – and many of their problems can be related to sugar metabolism or pancreatic disorders. They could suffer from severe migraines or headaches. Remember that the big toe is also the head reflex. Over the years, I have seen many cases of clients suffering from headaches who also had ingrown toenails. Check the section on meridians, and note which meridians run through the area of the foot where the physical deformities and problems are found, in order to ascertain which organ is faulty and needs correcting.

Plantar Digital Neuritis

Neuritis is the inflammation of a nerve, with pain, tenderness and loss of function. This particular form of neuritis affects the toes, usually the fourth toe. The pain usually begins at the web between the third and fourth toes and shoots up into the fourth toe. The sensations experienced in the toe may vary from slight numbness to intense pain, depending on how severely the nerve is affected. The discomfort can be alleviated by massaging the toe. This problem usually occurs in women.

Meridians and Plantar Digital Neuritis

The gall bladder meridian is found on the fourth toe, where this problem is most common. Plantar digital neuritis is found in many women, and I have witnessed numerous cases where women have this problem around premenstrual time when they often crave chocolates, caffeine and other stimulants. The condition can therefore be related to overloading of the gall bladder meridian. Often symptoms will indicate other gall bladder related problems. This can also be associated with hip trouble – and can possibly be seen as a puffy area in line with the fourth toe close to the ankle. The gall bladder meridian runs through the hip region, and swelling here may indicate congestions along the gall bladder meridian.

Flat Feet

Flat feet (Pes planus) can be caused by numerous factors. They are usually inherited, but may also develop due to weakness in the joints or 'overloading' the feet, or they may be the result of a long illness. In childhood this condition can occur if growth is too rapid, or if the child is malnourished or overweight. The weaker the foot, the greater the possibility of this condition developing. Apart from causing an unattractive style of walking, flat feet can also affect the spine.

In flat feet the arch of the foot is flattened and sinks. This causes overstretching and weakness of both muscles and tendons and places a strain on the bone structure. Another problem is that the nerves and blood vessels, which are usually protected from contact with the ground by the shape of the arch, are now subject to pressure and their condition will deteriorate affecting the reflexes in this area.

The Highly Arched Foot

The highly arched foot is usually stiff which limits manouvreability and therefore prevents efficient functioning of the foot. Due to the exaggerated height of the arch, the toes will not have correct contact with the ground when standing. The unnatural shape and position of the toes makes them particularly susceptible to external pressures and therefore prone to corns and callouses. This condition may be inherited or could be the result of nerve and muscle imbalance. It is often seen in the neurological conditions poliomyelitis and spina bifida.

As a reflexologist, I would see the problem of flat feet as related to a rigid spine, indicating that the person is not very supple and could also be inclined to lower back problems. A highly curved arch or curved spine reflex also indicates a spinal problem, and this can cause problems with the upper part of the body – the lung area. If you press your fist against the lung reflex of the foot and gently press the foot back into a normal position, you will see the spinal reflex 'correcting' itself, and can therefore deduce that the client has a tendency to lower back problems, neck tension, congestions in the lung area and, as the toes are often also affected, problems along the meridians found in the toes.

The Heel

As the heel is subject to immense stress and bears a great deal of body weight it has the extra protection of a thick layer of fatty tissue under the heel bone.

Heel Callous
This is formed when areas of skin around the edge of the heel become thicker than usual to protect it from aggravating pressure and friction. It can develop into a painful condition if not dealt with.

Heel Fissure
A heel fissure develops when the skin on the edge of the heel splits. This is usually due to the fact that the skin is excessively dry and is being pinched by ill-fitting shoes. If the fissure is deep, pain and bleeding can occur.

Reflexes/Meridians and Heel Problems
The heel is the pelvic reflex, and problems here will often indicate prostate problems in men and uterus problems in women. Many women have deep cracks in their heel just prior to a hysterectomy and these often heal naturally after a hysterectomy. Any other reproductive problems in men and women – infertility, heavy bleeding and discomfort – can be related to imbalances in the pelvic region. All six main meridians run through this area and organs and meridians can be stimulated by massage here.

6

Techniques

T HE BODY IS reflected on the feet in a three-dimensional form. In the body, the organs overlap each other; therefore the reflex areas do the same on the feet. Many organs are minute and not reflected on the charts, but all are worked on in the step-by-step treatment sequence. In the massage technique I teach, treatment always includes both feet. The reflex areas of both left and right feet are alternately massaged from toes to heel.

Many of the reflexology books available teach the 'thumb walking' technique and propose working one foot completely before moving on to the next. The main objective of the reflexologist is to stimulate the reflexes of the feet by massage. As any technique which achieves this result is equally effective, it is the prerogative of each individual practitioner to choose which technique works best for them. I have found in my years of practice and teaching that the techniques illustrated here have proven their worth for both practitioner and patient.

The most important aspect of this specific treatment procedure is that BOTH FEET ARE WORKED THROUGH ALTERNATELY FROM TOP TO TOE. This facilitates a natural flow in the procedure. One foot represents half a body, and as many organs are paired and found on both sides of the body, it would be wrong to complete one foot at a time. This would mean that only half the organ had been stimulated. The theory behind alternating feet is to stimulate each organ completely before moving on to the next. In this way each body part is worked as a unit even though half is on the left foot and half on the right. To execute effective reflexology massage techniques, familiarity with techniques and grips is a necessity.

Holding the Foot

Standard Support Grip (Figure 24)

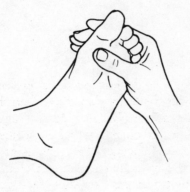

Fig. 24.

The first priority is to learn proper support or the pressure techniques will never be mastered correctly. The hands perform complementary functions throughout the treatment. While one hand presses, the other braces and supports or pushes the foot towards the pressure. To simplify things, the hand applying pressure will be referred to as the 'working hand' and the other hand the 'supporting hand'. Neither hand should ever be idle.

There is one main support technique. This is referred to as the *standard support grip* (Figure 24). Take the foot in the support hand, either from the inside or the outside – the web of the hand between the thumb and the index finger touching the side of the foot with the four fingers on top of the foot and the thumb on the sole. The support hand must always stay close to the working hand. Whichever grip you use on whatever reflex, always keep the foot bent slightly towards you and never in a tight grip with the toes bent backwards.

Pressure Techniques

The Rotating Thumb Technique (Figure 25)

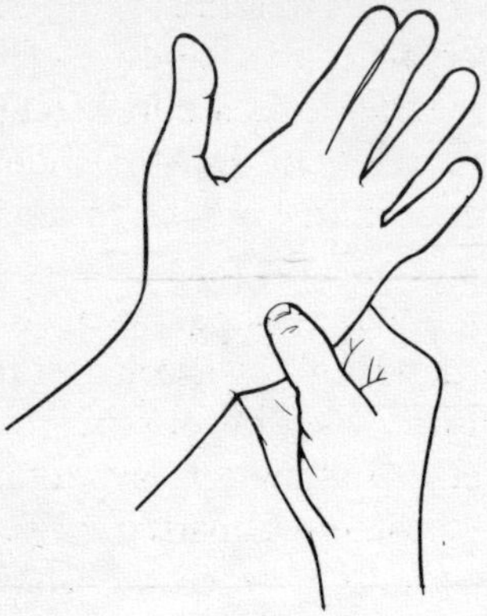

Fig. 25.

This is the most important technique to master, as it is used to apply pressure to most of the reflexes throughout the treatment procedure. It is combined with finger techniques.

Before working on the feet, exercise the 'rotating thumb' technique on the palm of your hand. It helps to visualize the object being worked on (hand or foot) as divided into small squares, all of which must be systematically stimulated. As you work, move from square to square, apply pressure and rotation to each square. The movement of the thumb from point to point must be small, moving along progressively, leaving no space between the points covered by the thumb tip.

For this exercise, place the four fingers of the working hand on the back of the hand to be worked on, keeping the thumb free to work on the palm. Bend the thumb from the first joint to between a 75 and 90 degree angle – the angle must ensure that the thumb nail doesn't dig into the flesh. This is the standard position of the 'rotating thumb'. The contact point is the tip of the thumb. Apply firm pressure with the tip of the thumb to the point to be worked on, and rotate the thumb, clockwise or anticlockwise. Keep the firm pressure constant and *stay on the square*. Two to three rotations are sufficient. Lift the thumb, move to the next point and repeat the procedure. The basic movement is: press in, rotate, lift, move. The choice to increase the amount of pressure or number of rotations depends on the practitioner and patient.

Observe the movement of the thumb on the working hand. The most visible rotation must be at the second thumb joint – where the metacarpals of the hand join the phalanges of the thumb. Two basic tenets for ease in executing this technique are to keep the thumb bent and the shoulders down. There should be very little strain on the arm muscles, elbows, neck and shoulders.

Furthermore, you will notice how much more pressure can be applied with the thumb in a bent position as opposed to a flat thumb. Ensure that the distance between the thumb and fist is sufficient to allow for easy rotation movements – approximately 2 centimetres apart. By exercising the correct technique, the treatment procedure should not be at all strenuous for the practitioner. Practise this thumb rotating technique on your hand until you feel completely comfortable with it. Also ensure that you exercise the thumbs on both hands to enable you to work efficiently with either thumb, as it is important to be able to switch hands during the treatment sequence.

Finger Techniques (Figures 26-28)
1. Hands are placed on either side of the foot with the thumbs on the sole and four fingers on top. The index and third fingers are the working tools, the third finger usually placed on top of the index finger to create extra leverage. This is used on the fallopian tubes/vas deferens and lymphatic reflexes which run

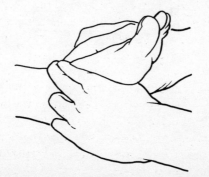

Fig. 26.

from the outside ankle bone along the top of the foot at the ankle joint to the inside ankle bone. With the fingers, press in, rotate, lift and move as with the 'rotating thumb', moving point by point up both sides until the fingers meet at the centre on top of the foot. (Figure 26)

2. This is used on the sides and tops of the toes. Place the index finger on one side and thumb on the other side of the

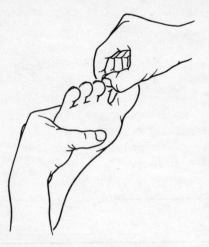

Fig. 27.

toe to be worked on. 'Rub' the toe, moving the fingers gently back and forth in opposite directions. (Figure 27)

3. Use both hands. Place the hands on either side of the foot, thumbs on the sole forming the support and four fingers on top.

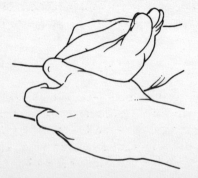

Fig. 28.

The eight fingers are the working tools. Starting from the ankle joint, exert deep, smooth pressure with the fingers massaging down the foot towards the toes – slowly and gently, but with firm pressure. Repeat this procedure a few times. Improvize a bit, but massage well. Also use a criss-cross movement with the thumbs on the sole of the foot. This is usually part of the winding down stage of the treatment which culminates in the solar plexus breathing technique. Cream or oil can be used at this stage to facilitate easy movement. (Figure 28)

Pinch Technique (Figure 29)

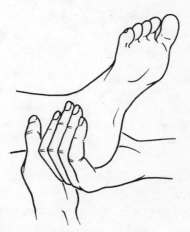

Fig. 29.

The support hand cups the foot at the ankle, while the working hand locates the tendon at the back of the heel and moves up and down the tendon pinching this tendon gently between the thumb and index finger. This is used to stimulate the kidney and bladder meridian.

Knead Technique (Figure 30)

This is a relatively easy technique, much like kneading bread. It is used mainly on the heel area which is usually rather tough, and therefore needs more pressure for effective stimulation. Cup the ankle in the palm of the support hand, keeping the heel area free. Make a fist with the working hand, then use

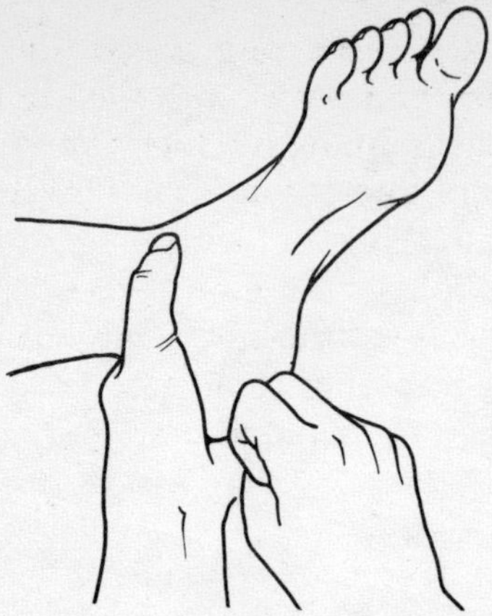

Fig. 30.

the knuckles of the second joint of the fingers to 'knead' the heel as you would dough. This is used for working reflexes in the heel – the sciatic reflex and nerve and the reproductive reflexes.

These are the main basic finger and thumb techniques used in the treatment procedure. As one of the main benefits of reflexology is the relaxation aspect, it is important to become familiar with a few basic relaxation techniques.

Relaxation Techniques

1. Achilles Tendon Stretch (Figure 31)
Cup the heel of one foot so that it rests in the palm of the hand. Grasp the top of the foot near the toes in the standard support

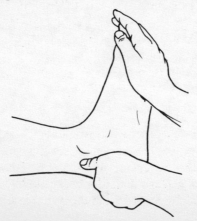

Fig. 31.

grip. Pull the top of the foot towards you, allowing the heel to move backwards, then reverse the procedure, pulling the heel towards you and pushing the top of the foot backwards so that the bottom of the foot stretches out. Repeat this two or three times.

2. *Ankle Rotation (Figure 32)*

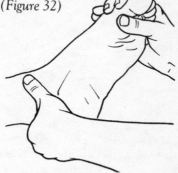

Fig. 32.

Cup the back of the ankle of the right foot in the palm of the left (support) hand, with the thumb on the outside of the ankle and the fingers on the inside. Ensure a firm but not tight grasp. Working with the right hand from the inside of the foot, grasp the foot at the base of the big toe in the standard support grip. Hold the foot with equal pressure. Use the hand holding the ankle joint as a pivot, and rotate the foot with the right hand in 360 degree circles, first clockwise a few times then anticlockwise. Work the other foot the same way alternating hands accordingly. Do not force the foot into exaggerated circles, manoeuvre it slowly and gently only as far as is comfortable for the client. This movement must be carried out smoothly and affects the entire area of the hip joint and tailbone, relaxes the anus and surrounding area and affects all the lower back muscles.

3. *Side to Side (Figure 33)*
This method of vigorously shaking the foot helps circulation, eases tenderness, and relaxes ankle and calf muscles. Place both palms on either side of the foot just above the ankles. Keep the hands as relaxed and loose as possible. Do not force the foot to rotate further than is comfortable for the subject.

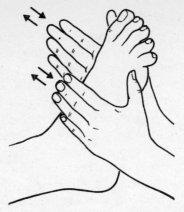

Fig. 33.

Roll the foot from side to side by gently moving it back and forth between your hands which move in opposite directions from each other. Move the hands gradually up the sides of the feet until the entire foot is worked. This is usually executed slowly to release tension, relax the edges of the ankle and calf and stimulate the whole foot.

4. *Loosen Ankles (Figure 34)*

Hook the base of both palms above the back sides of the heel so that the palms cover the ankle bones. The ankle joint serves as the pivot point. Move the hands rapidly backwards and forwards in opposite directions to each other, keeping the hands hooked beneath the ankle bones. The foot will shake from side to side when this movement is properly executed.

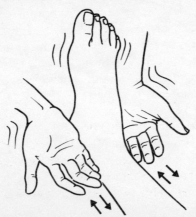

Fig. 34.

5. *The Spinal Twist (Figure 35)*
Grasp the foot from the inside of the instep with both hands, fingers on top, thumbs on the sole – the web between the thumb and the index finger on the spinal reflex. The index fingers of each hand should be touching. When working the right foot, the right hand starting position will be at the ankle joint on the top of the foot and vice versa on the left foot. The hand close to the ankle will provide the support. The hand nearest the toes will execute the twisting action. The two hands should be used as a unit, keeping all the fingers together and the two hands touching at all times. Keeping the support hand very steady, twist the working hand up and down. The support hand must remain completely stationary. Then move both hands forward slightly and repeat the twisting action.

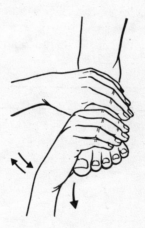

Fig. 35.

Continue this movement (grip, twist, reposition, grip, twist, reposition) until you reach the neck reflex area at the base of the big toe. Do not twist both hands at the same time. Repeat this on both feet. If the person is tense it may be necessary to repeat a few times. This is a very effective tension reducer, enjoyed by most.

6. *Wringing the Foot (Figure 36)*

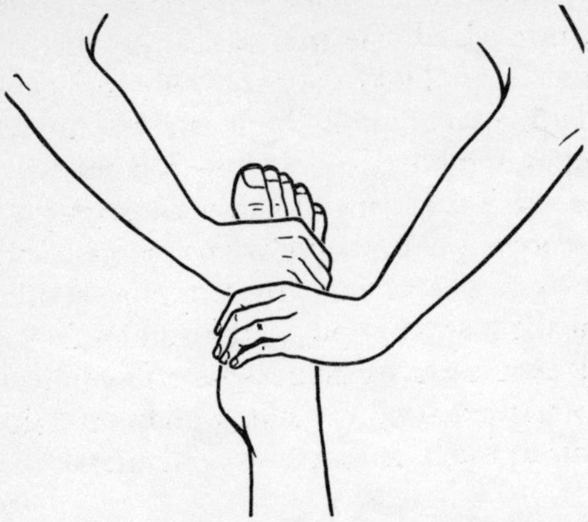

Fig. 36.

This is similar to the spinal twist, except both hands move in the wringing motion. Grab the foot in both hands as you would a wet towel and wring gently, each hand twisting in opposite directions. Your elbows should fly up and move when you do this. Move the hands gradually up the foot to 'wring' the entire foot..

7. *Rotate All Toes (Figure 37)*
The principle here is the same as the ankle rotation. It is a relaxation technique which not only increases flexibility of the toes, but releases tension and loosens muscles in the neck and shoulder line. The big toe is most important here. It represents half of the head area. The head joins the body as the toe joins

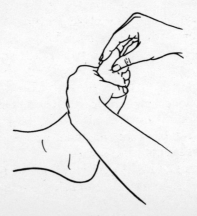

Fig. 37.

the foot, so the area joining the toe to the foot corresponds to the neck. To execute this procedure begin with the big toe and work through all the toes of one foot before moving on to the other foot. Hold the foot with the support hand in the standard support grip. With the thumb and fingers of the support hand, firmly hold the base of the toe you are going to rotate. With the working hand grasp the toe close to the base joint (metatarsal/phalange joint), with the thumb below, index and third finger on top. Now gently 'lift' the toe in its joint with a slight upward pull, and rotate in 360 degree circles, clockwise and anticlockwise a few times. Movements must be gentle but firm, the support hand stabilizing each toe individually at the base as it is worked on.

8. *Solar Plexus (Figure 38)*

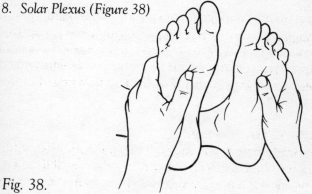

Fig. 38.

The solar plexus is referred to as the 'nerve switchboard' of the body, as it is the main storage area for stress. Applying pressure to this reflex will always bring about a feeling of relaxation. To locate the solar plexus reflex, grasp the top of the foot at the metatarsal area and squeeze gently. A depression will appear on the sole of the foot at the centre of the diaphragm line – the centre of the base of the ball of the foot. This is the solar plexus reflex. This technique is applied to both feet simultaneously. Pressure applied to this reflex is usually used as a relaxation technique to complete the treatment but can be used at any time during treatment if necessary.

Take the left foot in the right hand and the right foot in the left hand, fingers on top, thumbs below – from the outside of the foot. Place the tips of the thumbs on the solar plexus reflex. Ask the subject to inhale slowly as you press in on this point and exhale as you release pressure. Do not lose contact with the foot. Repeat this exercise a few times.

Grips

The following are descriptions of the specific 'hand-holds' (or hand positions) used in the practice of reflexology. They facilitate comfortable and effective execution of the thumb and finger pressure techniques.

Grip A (Figure 39)
Make a clenched fist with the working hand keeping the thumb free. The fist of the working hand will provide additional support on the sole of the foot. The 'rotating thumb' technique is used to exert pressure on the reflex points. The support hand is in the standard support position close to the working hand. With Grip A the left hand is usually the support hand and the right hand the worker.

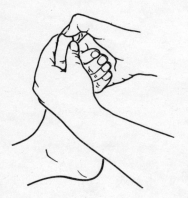

Fig. 39.

Reflexes worked with Grip A
Sinuses
Chronic eyes and ears
Bronchia, lungs, heart

Grip B (Figure 40)

Here the support hand holds the foot in the standard support grip close to the toes. With the working hand, clasp the foot from above. Place the fingers on the top of the feet pointing towards the ankle. The thumb is then positioned to work under the toes.

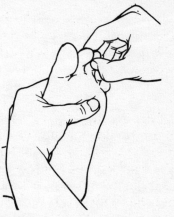

Fig. 40.

Reflexes worked with Grip B
Pituitary gland
Brain matter
Eyes and ears

Grip C (Figure 41)

This is an alternative grip with which to locate and stimulate the pituitary gland if you have trouble with Grip B. Bend the

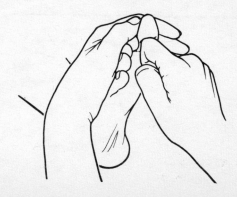

Fig. 41.

index finger at the second joint and use this as you would the thumb, find the reflex, press in, rotate clockwise and anticlockwise a few times then release pressure when you feel the reflex has been sufficiently stimulated.

Reflexes worked with Grip C
Pituitary gland

Grip D (Figure 42)
Here the left hand is the support hand and the right hand the working hand on both feet. 'Cup' the arch of the foot in the palm of the support hand. The thumb of the working hand provides extra support on the sole of the foot on the thoracic reflexes, and the index finger is responsible for the rotations on the top of the foot. Place the third finger on top of the index finger to enable you to exert greater pressure on the lymphatic reflexes. With the thumb on the sole and fingers on top, reach between the toes till the web between the thumb and index finger touches the web between the big and second toe. Reach as far down the top of the foot as possible with the fingers and, using the rotation movement as you would with the thumb, work point by point towards the webs. When you get to the webs, apply a tight, pinching pressure on the webs as these are the most active lymphatic reflexes. Repeat this between each toe, using the grooves between the metatarsal bones as guidelines. Repeat this procedure on both feet.

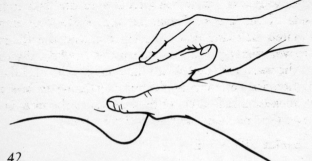

Fig. 42.

Reflexes worked with Grip D
Upper lymphatics

Grip E (Figure 43)
In this grip the elbows move out and up into the air to facilitate the angle necessary to get right into the thyroid reflex. The thyroid reflex covers the entire area of the ball of the foot at the base of the big toe, but the most important part of this reflex is found in the half circle shape right at the base of the ball, almost 'under' the bone. To achieve sufficient stimulation,

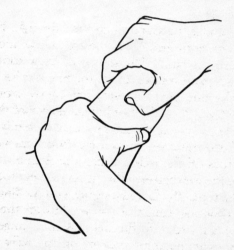

Fig. 43.

you must get right in to the bone at the base of the ball and press 'up and under'.

With the support hand, hold the foot in the standard support grip which must be positioned close to the working hand. The fingers of the working hand grasp the foot from the inside of the instep, fingers on top of the foot from approximately half way down the big toe, and the thumb poised to work the important half moon section of the thyroid reflex at the base of the ball. With the thumb, press in and up to get right to the bone and use the 'rotating thumb' technique to work round the half circle of the ball, up to the neck and then cover the section at the base of the big toe.

Reflexes worked with Grip E
Thyroid
Parathyroid
Neck

Grip F (Figures 44 and 45)
To execute this grip effectively, the practitioner must be seated in such a way as to be able to swivel in his/her seat so as not to be working the foot 'straight on'. When utilizing Grip F, always work the outside of the foot with the outer hand and support

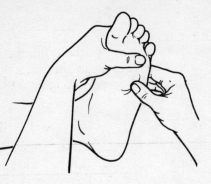

Fig. 44.

with the inner hand from the instep (Figure 44); and work the inner side of the foot with the inner hand from the instep and support with the outer hand (Figure 45). The pressure is, as usual, exerted with the 'rotating thumb'.

Imagine the foot divided in half vertically. The object is to work horizontally across both feet as if they are a single unit, using the imaginary vertical line as the point at which to swop working hands. This may sound slightly confusing at first, but it definitely facilitates a smooth and flowing technique for working the digestive area.

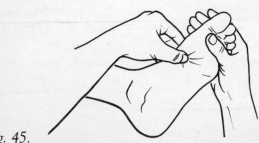

Fig. 45.

Reflexes worked by Grip F
Liver/gall bladder
Stomach, pancreas, duodenum, spleen
Small intestine, ileo-caecal valve, appendix
Large intestine
Kidneys, adrenals, ureters

Grip G (Figure 46)
For this grip, the foot is cupped in the palm of the working hand, the sole of the foot resting in the palm, leaving the thumb free to execute the 'rotating thumb' technique. The

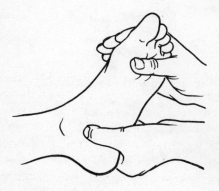

Fig. 46.

support hand is in the standard support grip. This grip is used mainly for working on the sides of the feet – the spine and bladder on the inner foot and the knee, hip, elbow and shoulder on the outer foot.

Reflexes worked by Grip G
Bladder
Uterus/prostate/ovaries/testes
Spine
Knee, hip, elbow, shoulder

STEP-BY-STEP TREATMENT SEQUENCE

The treatment sequence is divided into the same main areas as mentioned in Mapping the Feet (Chapter 4).

The Head and Neck Area – the Toes;

The Thoracic Area – the Ball;

The Abdominal Area – the Arch;

The Pelvic Area – the Heel;

The Reproductive Area – the Ankles;

The Spine – the Inner Foot;

The Outer Body – the Outer Foot;

Circulation – the Tops of the Feet.

Do not forget – the feet are worked alternately from toe to heel, organ by organ.

Easy Reference Treatment Procedure

This step-by-step sequence describes the various techniques and grips in the specific order which constitutes a full reflexology treatment. This is the standard sequence I teach, and I have found it gives optimum results.

Relaxation Techniques
Achilles Tendon Stretch
Ankle Rotation
Loosen Ankles
Side to Side
Wringing the Foot
Rotate all Toes

Head and Neck Area – The Toes
Sinus from big toe to small toe – Grip A
Pituitary gland – Grip B or C

Techniques

Brain matter – Grip B
Eyes and ears – Grip B
Sides and tops of toes – Finger Technique 2
Chronic eye and ear problems and eustachian tubes – Grip A
Upper lymphatics – Grip D

Thoracic Area – The Ball
Bronchia, lungs and heart – Grip A
Thyroid – Grip E moving to Grip A
Neck – Grip A

Abdominal Area – The Arch
Liver, gall bladder – Grip F
Stomach, pancreas, duodenum, spleen – Grip F
Small intestine, ileo-caecal valve, appendix – Grip F
Large intestine – Grip F
Kidney, ureter – Grip F.
Bladder – Grip G

Pelvic Area – The Heel
Pelvis and sciatica – Knead Technique

Reproductive Area – The Ankle
Prostate/ uterus/ovaries/testes – Grip G
Fallopian tubes/vas deferens – Finger Technique 1

The Spine – The Inner Foot
Spinal Twist – Relaxation Technique
Spine from heel to toe – Grip G

Outer Body – The Outer Foot
Knee, hip, elbow, shoulder – Grip G

Circulation/Lymphatics – The Top of the Foot
Lymphatics, breast area, circulation – Finger Technique 3

Relaxation Techniques
Kidney and bladder meridians – Pinch Technique
Solar Plexus Deep Breathing – Relaxation Technique.

7

Self-Help and Products

SELF-TREATMENT

SELF-TREATMENT WITH reflexology can be awkward and arduous, but if you are willing to devote the time and energy to yourself, it is certainly worth the effort. There are, however, disadvantages to self-treatment. First and foremost, all-important relaxation is impossible to achieve this way. And second, the vital energy exchange between subject and practitioner – which plays a major role in the success of treatment – is lacking, as you are both practitioner and patient at the same time. Self-treatment is therefore only useful as a means of preventative treatment, general health care and first aid treatment to achieve quick relief for a condition until you can arrange for professional treatment. It goes without saying that this form of treatment could never be as effective as a professional treatment from a trained practitioner.

However, for those who are willing and able to devote the time and energy to themselves, self-treatment can have beneficial results. It can be undertaken by anyone reasonably agile, who can comfortably sit cross-legged or raise a foot onto the opposite knee.

Comfortable seating is the first prerequisite. Sit on a chair, or cross-legged on the floor or bed with cushions behind your back. If you are aware which reflexes are out of balance, work specifically on those. If not, work calmly and gently through the whole treatment in accordance with the techniques and sequence described in Chapter 6. You should be as relaxed as possible with no tension in the legs. Remember it is difficult to assess your own reflexes accurately.

A full treatment will take approximately an hour, which may be a bit much for many to contemplate. However, treatment of appropriate reflex points can be used to relieve headaches, migraines, muscle aches and other transient conditions. At the end of a treatment, always take the time to sit or lie back for approximately fifteen minutes and relax with breathing techniques.

PRODUCTS

Creams and Oils

A therapist may apply herbal ointment or oil to stimulate circulation and relax the client at the end of a treatment. It is a good idea to pamper your feet like this at regular intervals – either after a self-treatment or merely to relax and revitalize your feet. There are numerous foot creams available on the market but it is preferable to use something herbal and natural, such as an aromatherapy oil or herbal cream, for their beneficial healing properties.

Foot Baths

Famous herbalist and healer, Maurice Messegue, recommended herbal foot baths as an essential part of his treatment. He believed treatment by osmosis to be most effective, as the main ingredients which contain the healing qualities of plants rapidly penetrate the skin and sometimes reach the affected areas more quickly than if the same ingredients are taken internally. He chose foot and hand baths over hip and total baths as they are easy to prepare and because the hands and feet are the most receptive parts of the body. These can be prepared with dried herbs or aromatherapy oils infused in boiling water. Foot baths should be taken as hot as possible (but not boiling) first thing in the morning on an empty stomach and should not last for more than eight minutes.

Chemical Foot Sprays
These should be avoided. They clog the pores and prevent the feet from being able to rid themselves and the body of excretions from the sweat glands. It is not wise to suppress the ability of the body to sweat through the feet. Excessive sweating is an indication of imbalance and should not be ignored.

Shoes, Socks and Stockings
Shoes, socks and stockings of synthetic materials should also be avoided as they increase the likelihood of sweating. Plastic and rubber shoes stifle the feet, while leather allows them to breathe. The same applies to nylon socks and stockings as opposed to cotton.

Reflexology Shoes
These shoes have 'quills' which massage the feet and stimulate the reflexes while walking. Using these is not a replacement for reflexology, but is beneficial in that they promote lymphatic drainage and circulation in the feet. These should only be used in moderation as exaggerated use can overstimulate reflexes and cause discomfort.

Other Foot Aids
There are numerous varieties of 'foot aid' available on the market today – reflexology mats similar to the shoes; wood or plastic rollers; brushes and electrically operated gadgets and all types of balls like golf and tennis balls are often recommended. As with the shoes, these help tone and relax the foot and increase lymphatic drainage and circulation but should only be used in moderation to avoid overstimulation. These are only effective for maintenance of good health, and not effective in treating specific problems. None of these aids can be more effective than, or can replace, professional treatment.

When using any of the 'roller' type aids, roll them in a uniform way with an even, light pressure over the entire foot – the bottom and sides of the feet. No special emphasis need be placed on any particular reflexes. Apply this rolling therapy every day for approximately ten minutes per foot.

It is important to remember that these implements give no clue to the differing state of tissue tone or allow for accurate reflex reading and reaction. Many practitioners would advise you to steer clear of them on the grounds that no mechanical implement could replace the practised hand of a practitioner for sensitivity. They can, however, be useful as preventative and maintenance therapy.

A natural foot massage is by far the best and is probably more effective than any gadget. A walk barefoot on the beach or the grass brings the feet into contact with the earth and the energies that flow through it, and provides a revitalizing, energizing and natural massage.

VacuFlex System
Modern technology's contribution to reflexology is the Vacu-Flex System. Laser technology is replacing the surgeon's scalpel; vacuum therapy and electrical stimulation makes acupuncture more comfortable. The VacuFlex System is a vacuum system which is modernizing reflexology. By applying pressure to the whole foot at the same time, the VacuFlex 'boots' stimulate all reflex areas in just five minutes. After removing the boots, discoloration of the corresponding reflex areas remains for a few moments, providing an accurate visual diagnostic aid. People generally find the boots less painful than hand massage and children can be treated quickly and comfortably with this system. This system also includes the treatment of acupuncture meridians, stimulating these with suction cups. So it is a two-in-one idea, reflexology and acupuncture. The entire treatment takes about half an hour.

FOOT CARE

Having now seen that every part of the foot represents a part of the body, the importance of treating the feet with care and kindness is obvious.

Regular washing and careful drying will prevent cracks developing. A pumice stone and creams help soften hardened areas. Problems such as corns, verrucas and athlete's foot should be dealt with and a chiropodist consulted for persistent problems.

Feet should be kept warm and comfortable at all times. There is a good reason for this. I am, at present, living in a warm, sub-tropical climate, and have numerous clients whose children suffer from runny noses, sinus and chest problems and bladder weaknesses. In this climate the temperature is usually high outdoors, so air conditioners are common. This results in constant movement between hot and cold conditions. Most children go barefoot, and a sudden drop in foot temperature affects the reflexes as well as the related organs.

A Case History

A young male client suffered constant sinus and chest problems and asthma attacks. He responded well to reflexology treatments, but there was a constant recurrence of asthma attacks and often a slight cold. I checked his daily routine. On rising in the morning he would go straight from the warm bed into the garden (onto the cool, dew-covered grass) to let out the dogs and collect his newspaper. He would then go back indoors for a shower and walk around barefoot on tiled floors. The rapid variations in temperature his feet were subjected to was having an effect on his entire body, causing this propensity to colds and asthma. I recommended that he wear shoes to keep his foot temperature constant and his condition improved tremendously.

REFLEXOLOGY AND OTHER THERAPIES

Reflexology is an extremely effective holistic therapy, the positive effects of which can only be further enhanced by any other holistic therapy, attitude and activity. Many different factors influence each individual and therefore his ability to assimilate and respond to the healing process. Numerous conditions have an effect on our being – some in our control, some beyond our control. In order to help offset the negative effects of conditions we cannot control such as the earth's gravity, the movement of the sun, moon and stars, global and social pressures, and climate, we should make more effort to alter those conditions we can change to make them work to our advantage. The things we can do for ourselves may require some discipline and effort, but will be a great contribution to acquiring perfect health. Those we can change are diet, relaxation and exercise.

One factor under our control which has a profound effect on health is diet. Many conditions cannot be treated 100 per cent effectively unless modifications are made in diet. A good practitioner will usually enquire about diet and make some useful suggestions.

Relaxation techniques will also be beneficial as an adjunct to reflexology treatment. These include Tai Ch'i, yoga, meditation, breathing and visualization techniques. Some form of more vigorous exercise such as aerobics, swimming, jogging and the like is also recommended.

As reflexology is a holistic therapy it can be effectively and successfully combined with various other holistic/natural therapies. These include Bach Flower Remedies, herbal treatment, naturopathy, ayurvedic medicine, homoeopathy, hydrotherapy, shiatsu or any other forms of massage, acupuncture and the Alexander technique to mention a few. However, all the different methods cannot be applied together, as too much stimulation will have adverse effects.

CONCLUSION

Reflexology is expanding rapidly throughout the world. This is evidence enough of its efficacy and popularity. The main objective of reflexology is to help people attain and maintain a better state of health and well-being. It does not promise to be a magic cure-all for all people and all ills. But there can be no question that reflexology has carved a respected niche in the realm of holistic healing techniques.

Man is far more than the sum of his parts. Reflexology helps us to attune to our bodies and understand ourselves as part of a greater whole . . . to tune in to the natural laws of the cosmos and work towards a more holistic approach to life, an approach that results in a balanced and fulfilled life.

Perfect health requires discipline and energy, but the effort pays good dividends. The choice is yours – a productive, peaceful and fulfilled existence, or a life riddled with pain, anger and disease. But remember the old yogi saying: 'Health is a responsibility.'

Bibliography

Byers, Dwight C. *Better Health with Foot Reflexology*, Ingham Publishing, 1983.

Connelly, Dianne M. PhD, M.Ac, *Traditional Acupuncture: The Law of the Five Elements*, 4th Edition, The Centre for Traditional Acupuncture Inc, Columbia, Maryland, 1989.

Gillanders, Ann. *Reflexology – The Ancient Answer to Modern Ailments* Gillanders, 1987.

Goosman-Legger, Astrid. *Zone Therapy Using Foot Massage*, C.W. Daniel Company Limited, 1983.

Gore, Anya. *Reflexology*, Optima, 1990.

Grinberg, Avi. *Holistic Reflexology*, Thorsons, 1989.

Hall, Nicola M. *Reflexology – A Patient's Guide*, Thorsons, 1986.

Hall, Nicola M. *Reflexology – A Way To Better Health*, Pan Books, 1988.

Ingham, Eunice D. *Stories The Feet Can Tell Thru Reflexology*, Ingham Publishing, 1938.

Ingham, Eunice D. *Stories The Feet Have Told Thru Reflexology*, Ingham Publishing, 1951.

Issel, Christine. *Reflexology: Art, Science and History*, New Frontier Publishing, 1990.

Kaptchuk, Ted J. *The Web That Has No Weaver*, Congdon & Weed, New York, 1983.

Kunz, Kevin and Barbara. *The Complete Guide to Foot Reflexology*, Thorsons, 1982.

MacDonald, Alexander. *Acupuncture – From Ancient Art to Modern Medicine*, Unwin, 1982.

Manaka, Yoshio M.D. and Urquhart, Ian A. PhD. *A Layman's Guide to Acupuncture*, Weatherhill, 1972.

Mann, Felix Dr. *Acupuncture*, Pan Books, 1971.

Marquardt, Hanne. *Reflex Zone Therapy of the Feet*, Thorsons, 1983.

Marsaa-Teegurden, Iona; *Handbook of Acupressure II*, Ginseng du Foundation, 1981.

Nightingale, Michael Dr *Acupuncture*, Optima, 1987.

Norman, Laura. *Feet First*, Simon & Schuster Inc., 1988.

Russel, Lewis and Hardy, Bob. *Healthy Feet*, Optima, 1988.

Thie, John F. *Touch For Health*, T.H. Enterprises, 1973.

Wagner, Franz PhD. *Reflex Zone Massage*, Thorsons, 1987.

Further Information

For further information on the International School of Reflexology and Meridian Therapy, and referrals to agents for Vacuflex Reflexology Systems, please contact:

Carol Bosiger
24 Benhurst Garden
SELSDON
Surrey CR2 8NS

Charmaine Christod
c/o M Hadges
24–22 86 St
Jackson Heights
NEW YORK 11369

Dr Moshe Becker
P O Box 2006
PETAH TIKVAH
49120 Israel

Ann-Chatrine Jonsson
Varmlandsvagen 438
123 48 FARSTA
Sweden

Lone Busch Hansen
c/o Ryttervanget 17
6400 SONDERBORG
Denmark

Andrea Schippers
Thuringerstrasse No 2
3430 WITZENHAUSEN 1
Germany

Inge Dougans
POBox 68283
Bryanston
Johannesburg
2021
South Africa

OTHER REFLEXOLOGY ASSOCIATIONS

Pennsylvania Reflexology Association
May Post
1900 Emerson Street
Philadelphia PA 19152
USA

Reflexology Research Project
Kevin and Barbara Kunz
PO Box 35820, Stn D
Albuquerque NM 87176
USA

Reflexology Association of Canada
Dan Bisson, President
PO Box 444
Richmond Hill
Ontario L4C 4YB
Canada

Association of Reflexologists
27 Old Gloucester Street
London WC1 3XX
England

Forenede Danske Zoneterapeuter
Chr Wintheravej 13
6000 Kolding
Denmark

International Council of Reflexologists
4311 Stockton Boulevard
Sacramento
California 95820
USA

For those who wish to pursue the study of reflexology further, Element Books publish The Art of Reflexology (a workbook) by Inge Dougans and Suzanne Ellis.

Index